between
angels &
demons

Emma Bowes Romanelli

NEXT CENTURY BOOKS

I

First published in the United Kingdom by Next Century Books Limited,
2004

Next Century Books Limited
P.O. Box 6113
Leighton Buzzard
Befordshire
ENGLAND LU7 0UW

www.nextcenturybooks.com

A CIP catalogue Record of this title is available from the British Library

ISBN 0-9544011-6-6

Printed in England by Butler & Tanner

Credits

Cover Design and Layout :
Funkbuddha

Illustrations by :
Jackie Astbury

Dedication

For Jeremy, Hannah, Timmy and William, who
held our world together.
And for Mummy and Daddy who built its
foundations on such solid ground.

Between Angels and Demons

By Emma Bowes Romanelli

Foreword by The Duchess of York

I first met Emma many years ago when she was receiving treatment for Lymphoblastic Leukaemia at Stoke Mandeville Hospital. I was instantly impressed with her humour and incredibly optimistic nature despite the fact that she was battling a potentially fatal illness which can kill within a matter of weeks. Through sheer determination, an unshakeable faith and with the extraordinary love and support of her family and friends, Emma survived the ravages of repeated chemotherapy and radiotherapy and triumphed over the disease.

'Between Angels and Demons' is Emma's remarkable story of her day-to-day battle with leukaemia. It is told with candour and honesty, and her endearing humour shines through the pages of this inspirational and moving book. Twelve years after she was told that she was dying, at the tender age of nineteen, Emma recalls the pain and suffering that she, and her parents were so cruelly forced to endure. But her indomitable spirit and deep belief that there was a future beyond the end of the world carried her through the devastating ordeal.

Emma's story is truly inspirational, deeply touching and will be a story that one will find is unforgettable.

I am delighted that Emma has so generously donated some of the proceeds from the sale of "Between Angels and Demons" to the Teenage Cancer Trust – a unique charity which cares for teenagers who are battling cancer.

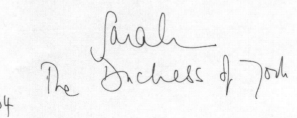

2004

V

'To see a world in a grain of sand
And a heaven in a wild flower
Hold infinity in the palm of your hand
And eternity in an hour...'

William Blake – 'The Auguries of Innocence'

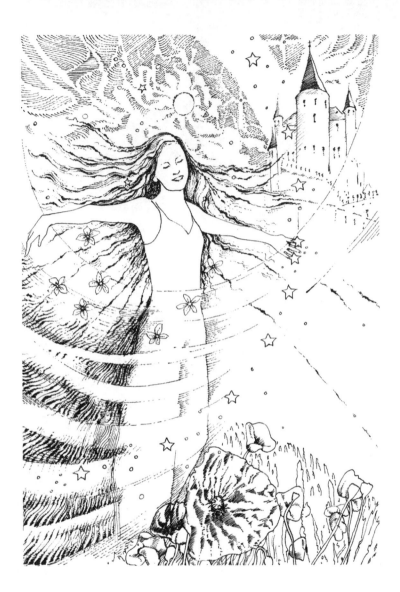

"...when your glass is always that full, you see, there is no room for the Bad Things."

Prologue

For some people, they say, the glass is always half empty. For others it is half full. Well mine is the glass that you have to pick up v-e-r-r-y slowly or risk it brimming eagerly over the edge in a wayward stream...And when your glass is always that full, you see, there is no room for the Bad Things. If they blow your way you let them drift on by, or kiss the frog to fairy prince, or dust the lining of the cloud with silver. But sometimes the Bad Thing is Really Bad and even if you screw it up very tight and small it is bigger than you are. And then the only thing to do is come out and fight. And all the time you are balancing that shining glass so precariously in your hands because you know that what you carry could not be more valuable if it were liquid gold. And all of a sudden you realise that that is what you are fighting for and that you would lay down your life for it because without your Spirit you have nothing and the Demons have won the war. And that can never be..........

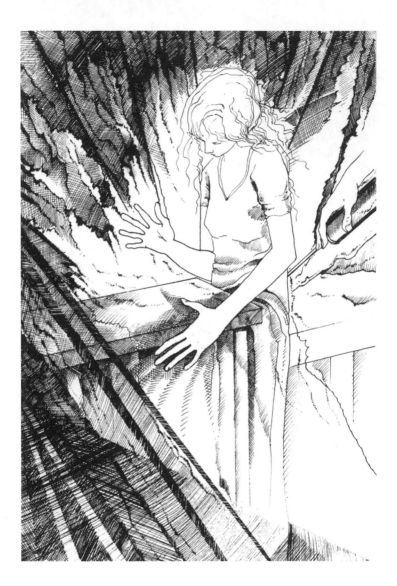

"My world ... confessed now to hidden, shadowy places..."

Chapter One
Dolly Mixtures

My first visit to Stoke Mandeville Hospital, some 15 years before, had been, in my opinion, a tremendous success. Not only did I clamber back into the car that fine December evening happy in the knowledge that I had a new, albeit rather crumpled, little sister, (Hannah), but, clutched proudly in my already sticky little fingers, was a large glass jar of Dolly Mixtures. Safely in Daddy's only marginally less sticky hands were the two glittery Christmas tree balls (proudly, if inexplicably, boasting the names 'Bruce' and 'Anthea' in homage to the presenters of the Generation Game!), that the nurses had also given my brother Jeremy and me in their general spirit of Christmas bonhomie. Suffice to say that where hospitals were concerned I was more than a little impressed.

Whilst my subsequent visits, (usually to A&E), had yielded less obvious fruit, they did generally facilitate a good few hours out of school and as such this early impression had stood the test of time.

Disappointingly then, at age 19, Ward 1X where we had been instructed to 'check in' was, to say the least, unprepossessing. A long, low construction, its appearance had rather more 'garden shed' about it than one might have expected given the hospital's reputation as one of the leading in the world. Nevertheless the warm, smiling faces of the staff did much to counteract this slightly gloomy air and I gave myself happily into the hands of the waiting doctor.

The first thing one could not help but notice about Dr O'Hara was her unruly cap of flaming red curls. The second was her soft, reassuring Irish accent and the third the gentle kindness in her twinkling green eyes. I liked her already. Leading us into a small side-room she gestured to me to sit down on the edge of the bed. They required me to answer one or two questions for their files before we began, she informed us, and Mummy nodded comprehendingly. I, on the other hand, went into paroxysms of anxiety. All was lost! She was bound to ask me about the contraceptive pill and with Mummy standing right there, wise, maternal and, above all… listening!! Such was my state of turmoil that I might have missed entirely God's timely, blessed intervention. "Perhaps you would rather we went through the questions in private?" the doctor inquired. "Your mother could wait outside the room for a minute." I nodded dumbly and looked shamefacedly across at Mummy. The door closed behind her and the confessional began.

A few minutes later, my ordeal over, Mummy came back into the room. Dr O'Hara looked kindly at us both. "We would like to run one or two tests just to confirm your previous results," she said. I nodded again and squeezed Mummy's hand. With that we were swept up into the hospital machine.
A gown arrived along with various items of medical paraphernalia, not least an extremely large syringe, and a number of young, smiley nurses. It was not until the doctor's next words, however that I began to feel just a little unnerved. "To ensure that you don't kick out with the pain," she explained, "we need to hold down this table across your legs. Try to keep as still as possible when the needle goes in." Hoping that my watery grin conveyed substantially more courage than I actually felt, I let them slip the hard, flat table over my legs and I bent forward over its cold, grey surface, revealing the base of

my spine for the needle. The next few moments - was it seconds, minutes or hours? – were indescribable.

The pain was of a kind that blacks out all other sensation, sight or sound. 'Do they realise,' my heart cried out in that dark, terrifying place, 'what they are asking me to bear in this? If so, then what else might they imagine I can endure and if not then surely there is no limit to what I might be subjected.' My world, only moments ago so safe and familiar, confessed now to hidden, shadowy places, sinister realms of uncertainty and fear beyond the reach of sun or reason.

I remember nothing of the transition from the shadows back to the crisp, white cool of the hospital bed. Mummy was still there beside me smiling reassuringly, drawing me back into the old world where the sun rises each morning and the sky goes on forever… Though I knew I would never forget where I had been, this was where I truly belonged and when Dr O'Hara slipped back into the room a few minutes later I greeted her, albeit in a necessarily horizontal manner, with the broad, triumphant smile of the survivor. She wondered if she could have a quick word with Mummy and I lay my head back down on the pillow, more gratefully, perhaps, than I might have admitted.

Not long afterwards she returned, this time without Mummy and I hoped with news of my test results. This particular adventure had not been as much fun as I had anticipated – there was not a Dolly Mixture to be seen - and I was, truth be known, more than ready to go home.

"Well," the doctor announced, "there is good news and bad news. Which would you like first?" Opting for the bad – it is always reassuring to know there is something coming to soften the blow – I waited patiently for her response; nothing could possibly be as bad as that infernal test, at any rate.

She hesitated: almost imperceptibly.

"The bad news is you have leukaemia. The good news is you have a 50:50 chance of living beyond the next few days…"

For an instant the world forgot how to turn. Then Reality and Reason got up and left the room.

The door banged shut behind them.

Chapter Two
Mr Roberts

When I was about nine years old I had a friend. His name was Mr Roberts and although there were probably more than 50 years between us we had one thing very much in common; a passion for writing. Once a week I would skip along the long winding road from home to call on him and his wife for tea. In the small cosy room beside the kitchen we would munch cake and reflect upon the week's events. Sometimes I would listen eagerly to tales of a world gone by; of secret bomb shelters under the stairs; of rationed bananas (in this respect, I surmised, their world of yesterday was not all that dissimilar to mine) and the crackling 'wireless'. At others they would sit smilingly and listen to my own tales, of bicycle picnics, school or my new baby brother. And then we would get down to business.

Mrs Roberts would briskly remove the tea tray and Mr Roberts and I would retire to the table. Spread neatly before us would be an early draft of the coming week's 'Wingrave Village Communiqué', of which he was the Editor. Rather more crumpled, my latest composition, be it poetry, book review or 'comment' would be held out for his revered opinion and hopeful inclusion in said esteemed publication.

When I grew up I was going to be a writer; I knew it and Mr Roberts knew it. I loved words. I loved the way they could be strong or gentle, light or dark; how they could transmute a scene or situation from sombre and threatening to gay and jaunty with just a few strokes of a pen. The power of language to linger lovingly over a long, languid summer's day or to give short, sharp shrift to the dank or dreary; to conjure the very essence of experience; image, sound, scent or feeling; through a well-chosen 'turn of phrase' was a continual fascination. Perhaps most of all I loved the way it could transport one to another here and now; to carry one to another world far beyond the confines of this but close-by enough for one to return home in time for tea.

When words become language, then they call out for a reader. Sometimes it might be just one but at others it needs to be shared by many to fully find its voice. Publication. This was where Mr Roberts came in. Week after week his gentle, wise encouragement and his unfailing ability to confer with me not as adult to child but as equals saw me tripping excitedly along the grassy bank from home, latest composition in hand, knowing that this was just the beginning...

Then, all of a sudden, it wasn't.

From the moment Mrs Roberts opened the door I knew that there was something different about this week. "You can't stay today," she informed me in an unfamiliar, brittle tone and I felt the already dark, cold entrance hall shudder.

"Can I just give this to Mr Roberts?" I asked hopefully, holding out that week's offering.

"Mr Roberts is ill," she replied, ignoring the paper thrust before her. "Go home. You mustn't come for a while."

"Couldn't I just say hello?" I pushed, sad to hear that my friend was sick.

Just then came the almost ethereal tinkling of a little bell.

16

Mrs Roberts cast her eyes up the narrow staircase. "Now see what you have done, you have disturbed him," she muttered accusingly. "Go home."

Just for a moment I too glanced up the stairs, fancying I was sending get-well messengers up to the unseen bedroom beyond; then I turned, mumbled my goodbyes and set off for home.

I never saw Mr Roberts again. One day he was there; forever afterwards he is the momentary tinkling of a little bell.

It was cancer that got him.

Chapter Three

Prognosis

It wasn't going to get me.

Chapter Four
Initiation

The first two weeks, my doctors had informed us, would be a kind of 'drug initiation' period, before the real stuff began.

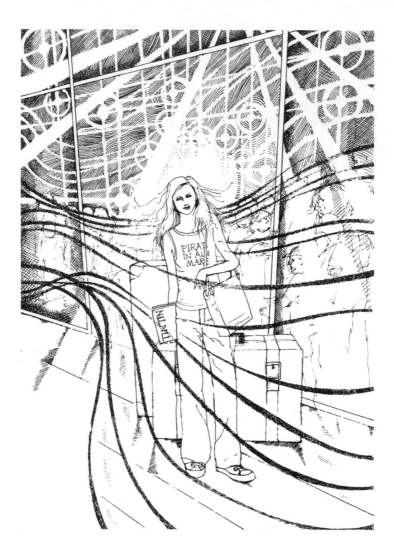

"I skipped, joyfully unburdened, into the arrivals hall."

Chapter Five
Pirates on the High Seas

My hand-luggage had consisted of two Tintin books, the most favoured of my vast Teddy-Bear collection and about four pounds of, it later transpired, illegally-smuggled Granny Smith apples. If the US film industry – and my determinedly English father – were to be trusted, there was not much call for fruit in this God-forsaken land of Burgers and Coke and I, for one, was determined to delay the onset of scurvy for as long as possible.

I had not been much reassured to learn from a friendly fellow passenger that TWA, (who were supplying my wings on this first, momentous flight of independence), (allegedly!) recycled the cast-off planes of other, less irresponsible airlines, but hey! I was striking a blow for freedom, no rusty tail-fin was going to cramp my style! Having spent the previous month and a half earning the approval of my parents (and having a fascinating and fun few weeks, it is only fair to add), working for an Art Gallery in Gloucestershire, I was now set to spend the next twelve months in the good old US of A!

There's no doubt that there are more Romantic, adventurous, scenic or exotic places in which to start out on the road to life but I had to agree with my 'elders and wisers' that as an 18 year-old blonde, whose most challenging experience to date had been the inadvertent breaking of a well manicured fingernail, I was perhaps not ready for the lone trek in the Himalayas that my soul was calling out for... Lara Croft I am not and, though it offends my poetic sensibilities to admit it, I have never been a 'roughing it' kind of girl. Remote, crashing waterfalls, bare-back riding across a Mongolian plain, cheek-by-jowl observation of the feeding habits of the wild Mountain gorilla – just try to hold me back – but when it comes to peas under the mattress, I am, most definitely, a Real Princess.

With both my father and I being equally excited by the idea of my financial independence, a 'working holiday', within the bosom of a family almost as large as my own, was ideal. Though to some the prospect of watching over four children between the ages of three months and seven years whilst their mother flitted from baby-shower to shopping mall may well rank among the most life-threatening experiences they are ever likely to avoid at all costs, I had been doing much the same thing (only with the mother, mine, and without the baby-showers) for as long as I could remember. Or so I thought. Interestingly that seemingly minor distinction, 'with the mother', counts for rather more points than one might credit but at this early stage, reclining in blissful ignorance in my TWA lounger, all was very much right with the world...

Five hours or so later, (and four pounds of – confiscated – illegal apples lighter), I took my first steps on US soil – or, to be uncharacteristically pedantic, tarmac. Fortunately still without a criminal record (see 'apples') and, less fortunately, also minus one Tintin book which had proved irresistible reading for the well-meaning, if somewhat negative, (see 'rusty tail-fin') couple who had peered sideways over my shoulder throughout the trip, I skipped, joyfully unburdened, into the arrivals hall.

My first impressions of JFK airport were of Big, Bright and Bustling with only the merest hint of Lonely. The sunlight poured in through the glass doors and with it a myriad of faces that, unlike the sun, poured out again with equal purpose. My year's worth of luggage proving somewhat burdensome, I opted for the composed, if not to say static, approach to exploring my surroundings, the constant tide parting and breaking only momentarily as it flowed by. The minute, and entirely inexplicable, Italian phrase which adorned my chest, 'Pirati in Alto Mare' (Or, 'Pirates on the High Seas', a minor designer-label T-shirt, financed courtesy of aforementioned gallery in Glos) took on new-found poeticism as I met each wave with stoic, territorial pride - though any faint echo of menace or cynicism was, undoubtedly, thoroughly quashed by the gleaming, pastel-coloured, baseball boots which I sported with equal élan. (Well, one never knows when one might be called upon to leap eight feet into the air and drop a ball into an unfeasibly small hole – stylishly). Anyway, fortunately, just as one or two of the circling sharks were beginning to take a somewhat predatory interest, I was wrested from my dramatic reverie by the sound of my name…

The last time I had seen Arabella was in the school library. Her head bowed, Arabella was bathed, angelically, in the kind of studious glow that, ordinarily, teachers can only dream of. My own aura I can only confess to being of a more abstracted nature, projecting, equally profoundly, the enviable if a little too complacent status of Lower, as opposed to Upper, Sixth. Whilst Arabella had just entered the Last-Chance Saloon where A-levels were concerned, I still had many reckless months of procrastination ahead and determined to allow my spirit and imagination free, unfettered reign with which to make the most of them. Strangely, then, her diligent absorption was almost enviable – such intensity of focus touched in me that passion for learning and discovery which I had allowed to fade in the face of competition from the splendid emotional excesses of teenage life.

Almost exactly a year later, once again in the library – fitting, since Arabella, I believe, had been its 'monitor' – I was to recall this gentle intellectual prod. We all sat cross-legged and cross at the end of another long and, in our present exam-wracked mode, irrelevant assembly as the Head of Upper Sixth read Arabella's letter aloud. Her animated account of her year 'stateside', with its 'This Could Be You Too' subtext, resounded through the room and once again Arabella's life nudged mine as, while I listened, the seeds of my adventure began to grow...

The journey from letter to The Big Apple, via the not insignificant hurdle of those pesky exams, was astonishingly swift and trauma-free. My father rallied magnificently after his initial horror (apocalyptic mutterings about strangulated vowels, chewing gum and baseball caps and the odd damning allusion to my forgoing any future rights to civilised society), even to the extent of forwarding the necessary funds for my flight. This benevolence though was on condition of full reimbursement on my return, laden down, as I would be, by the glittering fruits of my labour (a common and highly optimistic delusion, characteristic of the (usually male) parent of the species). Admittedly last minute disaster loomed when, in the heat of the emotion, we missed the turn-off for Terminal 1, but, it seemed, fate was not to be thwarted, even by an endless dual-carriageway going the wrong way. Nevertheless, the sight of Arabella's beaming face in amongst the pirates was a hugely reassuring one. Letters and phone calls are all very well but there is nothing like a friendly, exceedingly tangible, hug to persuade one that everything is going according to plan.

She was to have two weeks in which to 'show me the

ropes' before abandoning me to my own devices. I had, it seemed, a lot to live up to. Arabella was truly "one of the family" and they were all going to "miss her terribly".

In applying through our school, the Colcannon family were hoping to find "a girl just like her" and, I was horribly afraid, this was not altogether what they were getting. Whilst I undoubtedly had all the right intentions, Arabella, even on my brief, invariably library-bound glimpses, had the air of someone who had been designated 'monitor', 'prefect' or just plain 'in charge' of everything she had come into contact with since the year dot. Even the seemingly indestructible school geraniums had died when given over to my charge. The overwhelming impression I had gleaned from our correspondence was that of a shy, warm-hearted 'homebody' for whom this experience was merely the prelude to a more official future in the same vein. Though I like, of course, to think of myself as warm-hearted, here the similarity drew to an extremely decided close as far as I could see. For me the cosy nucleus of the family had already taken on vast, if not to say, global potential in terms of my introduction to the Big, Wide World. I would give my 'all', as is my wont, to the family and the challenge ahead but there would be plenty more 'all' to spare with which to discover and explore as much of life and the world 'without' as was in-humanly possible..!

My first sight of Arabella, 'stateside', then, was particularly reassuring. The open, confident girl that stood before me radiated the kind of liberated happiness that comes with the newly-found understanding and, perhaps, acceptance of oneself. Her hair radically cropped and her body language entirely altered, Arabella was powerful testimony to an altogether more positive, and equally pervasive, influence of the American Culture than that which kept my father awake at night. (Granted he could have won back a few points via the ubiquitous baseball cap, jeans and outsized T-shirt that had replaced the sensible shoes and pinafore dress of old, but with his own daughter sporting such a natty pair of pink baseball boots he might have done just as well in keeping quiet!)

All this boded well and, as we stepped out of purgatory into the warm, new light, I could feel the rest of my life beckoning me on…

Chapter Four Reprise
Initiation continued.....

Like the three wise monkeys, they had stood in white-coated, sensible-skirted triplicate at the foot of my bed, Drs O'Hara, Siskin and Watkins, as they doled out my fate.

After this time I would be very sick; indeed if the disease itself did not get me then the treatment might well do so. Up until then I could host friends and family freely, could have flowers in my room, still belonged in part to the world outside; afterwards I belonged to them. I nodded in pretence of comprehension, and thus, like Faustus with the devil, I made the pact.

Chapter Six
'Lights, Camera, Action'...and Cheese Puffs

Climbing up into the big, red 'family-cruiser' was more than a little like stepping into a film set. I have never been able to concur with the opinion that films are not true to real life as they are too implausible. Frankly, with each year that goes by my life becomes increasingly, staggeringly implausible. In fact I would challenge any scriptwriter to come up with a plot even remotely as unlikely as my own... Anyway, at this point I was marvelling in the realisation that American life, as per a zillion Hollywood re-makes, really...,well..., is. In addition, the overwhelming smell of 'cheese puffs', which seemed to cast a lurid orange, utterly un-cheese-like, glow over all, was beginning to ring my scurvy alarm bells in a truly alarming way. Lord Nelson thought he had problems on the HMS Victory but at least he didn't have to contend with cheese puffs... Through the orange haze I could dimly make out four bodies of varying diminutive stature, the sound emanating from which was decidedly not relative. Though their fingers were a different colour to that alluded to in my brief, (namely orange), the remaining distinguishing features seemed to confirm that here, in all their 'Parenting' glory (where is Steve Martin when you finally need him?), were indeed Patrick (aka 'Patch'), aged seven; Caroline, three (and a very important half); Victoria (fondly known as 'Tory'), two; and Catherine, three months and blessedly too small for cheese puffs, (even in Hollywood). Said occupants could not have been less moved by my arrival if they tried. Had I been bearing something of the wheat/ potato/ cholesterol snack variety I might at least have caused a stir, but, as it was, I didn't. Fortunately their mother was rather more forthcoming. A tiny red-head with curls that were even more bubbly than she was and a penchant for cheese puffs which made the continual diets rather hard to adhere to, her broad smile could not have been more welcoming. No doubt her relief at having Arabella back in the car, along with reinforcements, did much to enhance her mood but nevertheless as a temporary boss and, if my cards were on the table, surrogate mother for the coming year, she could not have been more reassuring.

All that remained then was the ceremonial parting of the crisp packets as I squeezed myself on to the spacious but already bulging magic carpet and we were off...

Destination: Marblehead, Massachusetts, a small harbour town on the East Coast, via a few bites out of 'The Big Apple' itself! To hit New York, New York whilst still dripping from my spate in the deep end was more than a little surreal. I was beginning to feel that 'Mom' ("Mo-aaaaaaaaarm") Colcannon had been at least mildly calculating in her suggestion of my personal limo service from JFK back to base. There is nothing like a few hours spent locked in a 'family-cruiser' to get to know your neighbours on an intimate basis. This nowhere-to-run method had ensured that, by the time we pulled up outside the Sheraton Hotel, introductions had been well and truly made and firmly, if a little greasily, cemented over a symbolic cheese puff or two.

The wood-panelled luxury of our home for the night was an indulgent if anachronistic introduction to the modern splendour that is Manhattan. A hop and a skip (I knew those baseball boots would come in handy!) from the

Empire State Building, we were perfectly based to make a speedy tour of the sights before cocooning ourselves in crisp linen and the soothing arms of sleep. Well, this was the theory. Always two steps ahead of reality in my burgeoning, optimistic imagination, I am increasingly aware of a recurring necessity to back-edit my original take on a situation from the marginally cooler light of day. In this case the temperature was lowered a good few degrees with the revelation that we were all to share a room. (SHARE A ROOM!). The fact that there were seven of us and there was only one (admittedly large) bed paled dramatically into insignificance when up against the fact that four of these were misogynistic megaphones with orange hands. Still, ever one to find that hint of silver in even the most lurid of clouds, I had to concede that they were at least small and this was definitely one of those times when size mattered. Nevertheless, not quite as captivated by the idea of TV and (YET MORE!) cheeselets as our room-mates appeared to be as we closed the door behind us, it was with glee and a certain amount of relief that Arabella and I leapt upon the suggestion to stretch our legs…

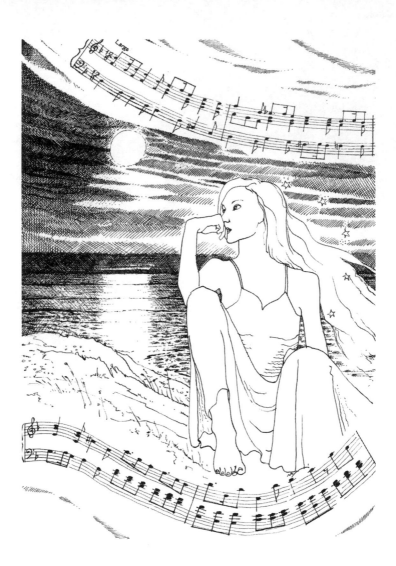

"...a perfect memory of freedom and joy".

Chapter Seven
Parenthood

That first night in America, with its whistle stop introduction to the sights and sounds of a whole new world, saw, in a blaze of lights and the roar of the crowds, my childhood step down, making way for the eager, if green, ascension of young adulthood. From that time on, how quickly I acclimatised to the after all not so alien culture that steals ever more hungrily across our own, is perhaps testimony to the extraordinary adaptability of human kind and the natural instinct of the young to strike out and forge their own individual path in the world.

Though only weeks before I had been frantically condensing the entire historical landscape of 16th and 17th century Britain and Europe into a small Rymans box-file, (pausing periodically for the cathartic slamming of numerous doors in order to convey to all in earshot the full burden of such a task), I was, before you had time to say 'supercalifragalisticexpialidocious', giving Mary Poppins a darn good run for her money. Where at home the opening of a tin of cat food (how it STINKS!!) was indisputable testimony to the immense love I had for my cat, here I found myself forging intimate (and entirely indiscriminate) relations with the putrid, rank and altogether vile without so much as a pause for thought.
 Another day, another teaspoon down the slimy, man-eating garbage disposal. One warmed bottle of milk in = one weighty 'diaper' out. In retrospect, in fact, the daily routine was characterised to a remarkable extent by things going in one end and appearing from another in a dramatically modified form, the latter, more often than not, distinctly unsavoury. Though the old me was

not, admittedly, altogether vanquished – why all mothers don't switch to wearing their bikini for the daily chores after the fifteenth outfit suffers the permanent indignity of baby-sick stains across the shoulder is beyond me – the new me was determinedly rising to the challenge.

Increasingly, though, I marvel at the reckless abandon with which the Colcannons senior handed over their offspring to an eighteen year old dreamer with pink and blue baseball boots and a matching bikini, but abandon them they did. For Mrs C., celebrating the liberation from pregnancy appeared to involve putting as much distance between herself and the fruits of her labour as possible – on a daily basis. Mr C. , though the amiable, baseball-cap wearing lawyer father beloved of many a Hollywood director, showed a distinct lack of Steve Martin's prowess in the entertaining department and timed his returns of an evening perfectly for the goodnight kiss on a peachy-clean cheek. (That of the babes in arms, as opposed to mine, it is important and not, I understand from other young 'nannies', altogether gratuitous, to add). Where would he be when they really needed him? – standing shivering, for example, outside an illegally-entered nightclub at 2am having missed the last train home..? (My Father, the hero!). Doubtless 'Patch' is now putting him to the test.

Anyway, even to me my eagerly claimed credentials for the job were debatable. Certainly, as the eldest of five children, I had had more than average experience in the babysitting department and my negotiating skills were legendary. I was generally the one called upon when my youngest brother, when aged six, had an attack of manic depression/ melodrama (understanding as I did the need to live permanently on the 'emotional edge') but I have no doubt that Jeremy, next in line after me, could testify to a number of occasions when his acute melancholy

could (ALLEGEDLY) have been attributable to yours truly. Sure, I had undoubtedly smelt a good deal of nappies in my time, but I was as likely to be found actually changing one as I was conceding defeat in a game of, well, anything…(despite, ye- s, ye-s, 'being the eldest').
I was, of course, quite happy to be a voluntary member of the entertainments committee – who ever tires of making 'play-dough' animals or chocolate rice-crispie cakes? – but prising a hysterical two-year-old off the swings when it was time to go home was generally beyond the bounds of my benevolence. Frankly though, it seems to me, the distinction between the roles of 'Big Sister' and 'Mother' is most neatly outlined in terms of how many people you are obliged to take with you to the 'bathroom'. Hitherto, I confess, I had been blissfully unaware of the air of decadence surrounding making this a solo venture. Maintaining one's dignity whilst juggling one member of the audience under each arm and finishing chapter seven for a third is, I can tell you, no mean feat. The calls of duty and nature do not, take it from me, go readily hand in hand. Nevertheless we made the best of it and, come to think of it, since when I didn't need to go someone else invariably did, we whiled away many companionable hours squeezing in and out of the 'little-ist room'. Nowadays I feel positively lonely.

Responsibility is a word that looms large in the world of the eldest child. Whether aged 3, 10, 15 or 25, you are always the one who 'ought to know better', 'should set a good example' AND has to feed the rabbits. Thus my inner child, though undeniably more resonant than most, sits ironically alongside a sense that I have been 'grown up' since shortly after I could walk. Historically, such 'precociousness' – particularly before I had reached double figures –did little to endear me to 'grown ups' of more advanced years but there was no doubt that here it was to truly come into its own. My awareness that in my charge were four new canvases, small sponges unconsciously programmed to absorb my every word and gesture in the process of forming their own blueprint on life, brought with it the enormous burden of conscience and no small degree of panic. Germinating minds, it seemed, had the unnerving ability to transpose one's pearls of wisdom into something altogether more hair-raising, before one had time to catch breath. One might even go for days with the naive glow of self-satisfaction that the data had been correctly processed, only to be cruelly stripped of one's illusion further down the line.

Tory, at two and a half, was particularly proficient in this art of 'wrong-footing'. How warm and beneficent I felt following an unfortunate incident involving the cream wool sofa and a large cup of orange juice. How I would have advanced Tory's journey to complete adult-hood in the calm, reassuring but firm way that I engaged her in the extensive clean-up operation. How my enthusiastic praise as she wielded the cloth would guide her on the straight and narrow path of those who do not allow that brief but fatal lapse of concentration when wielding their mid-morning tipple. How wrong I was. Too late I recalled the wisdom of 'Epaminondos', the cautionary tale of the wise mother whose loving, forgiving praise for her son's 'owning up' to breaking a plate resulted in his subsequently demolishing the entire house in the beaming anticipation of pleasing her. The tale had seemed quite a riot as a child but, as I, one fine morning, confronted the reality of Tory, dish-cloth in one hand, rapidly emptying juice cup in the other, the boot was very clearly on an altogether less tickled foot. "Good job, good job", Tory beamed back at me, in a familiarly reassuring and enthusiastic tone as she continued her jaunty alternation between 'spilling' and 'wiping' and I crossed teaching off my hypothetical list of career possibilities…

My responsibilities, it seemed, knew no bounds, ranging from moral to mortal (an episode with a large – and clearly carnivorous - hornet that Patch saw as essential to his collection of large and lethal insects of all kinds springs to mind), pausing to dwell upon embarrassing along the way. Who could have foreseen that the moment that Supergirl (guess who?) was triumphantly saving the Universe, not only single-handed but, (with the aid of an opportune climbing-frame), upside-down to boot, would coincide so anguishingly with the discovery that whilst in England lawnmowers tend to be squat and green and run on petrol, those in America are 6ft 2", blond, run on Nachos and are a good deal more stealthy in their approach? Still, it is, as they say, all part of the learning experience and you can be sure that the next time I am saving the Universe, I will be wearing my best knickers…

It was, however, a glorious summer. As each day the new- morning sun streamed across the harbour and in through the windows of my little attic bedroom, I had never felt more alive. For the first time I was creating my own story; author as well as protagonist. My fate was now in my hands, no longer in the charge of the ghost-writers; parents, teachers, 'the system'. With this recognition came a thrill of excitement, perhaps a little tinged with fear, but nothing was going to hold me back from taking hold of life with both hands; of inking each and every blank page that now called out so enticingly for my pen. Ideally, the year that stretched ahead, with a deferred university place comfortably awaiting my return home, afforded the perfect platform from which to embark on this first solo flight. In a sense it offered a unique 'window of independence', the illusion of freedom with all the security of the old establishment hiding in the wings. Here I could take my first shaky steps, safe in the knowledge of the familiar, strong hands waiting to catch me if I fell.

And take them I did. Skipping along to the nearby beach; running hopefully behind the Boston bus; dashing to make the early-evening performance at the local cinema or climbing up the grassy hillside above the ocean to catch the other-worldly strains of the little string quartet that serenaded the sun as it slid majestically behind the waves; this became my world, my story; one of sights, sounds, scents and tastes that will remain within forever, distilled into a perfect memory of freedom and joy.

But I couldn't ignore the 'tugs'. Mrs C. was wise to them, perhaps even before myself. I wasn't, as I was all too aware, (see 'geraniums'!), Arabella. For me there existed a whole inner world that craved attention and stimulation, a world that indulged wholeheartedly in a well-earned hiatus but one which, as time passed, threatened to strain yearningly at the bounds of a long, harsh New England winter. As the exciting newness of experience gave way to routine familiarity and an increasingly housebound existence, I would, she feared, become bored. Still bathed in the golden glow of summer, I countered her fears; in any case I had pledged to stay for a year and I was not about to abandon my post. In contemplative moments, however, my mind toyed disquietingly with her words, tantalised too by the offer of a position at the art gallery, should I decide to return home. Physically and mentally exhausted by 7.30 each evening, I had found myself retiring to bed increasingly early, unable to celebrate my freedom from duty with anything other than a restorative night's sleep in preparation for the next shift. Was this really the most fulfilling, and therefore prudent, use of this valuable year? Still, I resisted temptation, stoically deflecting the continual emotional pressure of my abandoned boyfriend across the sea and immersing myself in all that was positive about the 'here and now'. Until, that is, that fateful phone call.

Chapter Four Reprise
Initiation continued....

The doctors' voices were muffled somewhat by the wall that grew up daily between me and the unnatural, incomprehensible world, of which, to the uninitiated, it might appear I was now a part. Still, they went on to explain the structure of the following few years – were I, that is, to survive them. The odds, they said, were not good.

Chapter Eight

Miracles

Surprisingly, it wasn't the A grade in English Language and Literature, or the B in Art and Art History (that wretched still-life paper!) that inspired my whoops of joyful disbelief as I relayed the news to my parents but the, I knew sorely undeserved, C in History. Those last-minute relations with the Rymans box-file and the desperate, ink-stained companionship of my friend and fellow-procrastinator Kate, had, it seemed paid off. As the telephone and I danced our celebratory dance, so the mighty door between school and the 'real world' clanged shut. In the tale of 'my life' this was what my long-suffering history tutor would call a 'watershed', a pivotal point from which an Empire would rise or fall; one from which my entire future would find direction. Ironically, the knowledge that my university place at Leicester to read English and History of Art was secure, that I was steering nicely into the next port of call, led me rather to question how surely I wanted to dock. Instead of consolidating my future, the news brought with it the hazy cloud of uncertainty. Where Leicester was concerned, I realised, it came down to passion. There simply wasn't any. From my first interviews I had really just been going through the motions, setting up the next rung of the ladder. Could I knowingly resolve to embark down any future path without the spring of passion in my step? My new, adult ego jostled with the child. Surely the decision had been made? Could I challenge the accepted path? ...... Again the gallery's offer of a permanent position, a forerunner in their new London-based enterprise, skipped flirtatiously into view. If I returned home now, I had time to give the job a trial before making a final decision… There were definite echoes of those books or computer games that lead one merrily into a fantasy wilderness, place a dragon on the path to one's left ("turn to page 14"), a troll on the path to one's right ("turn to page 18") and then leave one to choose which way to go, facing the music accordingly. Fortunately in this case neither of my options was likely to lead to my ("hard fought") untimely demise but nevertheless my position was a daunting one. And this time I couldn't just shut the book and go and play in the garden instead.

In my anguish of indecision, (who'd be an author anyway?!), I turned, as I had always done as a child, to the ultimate Editor-in-the Clouds, God.

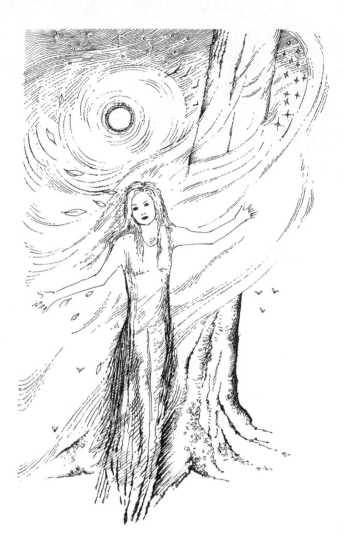

"Sometimes when I feel the wind on my face I know that God is speaking to me..."

Chapter Nine

God

My relationship with God is not altogether a conventional one. For as long as I can remember (and I suspect a good many millennia before that), He has simply always been there. There are possibly those, particularly of the Catholic persuasion, (I have a feeling that, in the Church of England, pretty much anything goes nowadays – Henry would surely be delighted!), who might feel my demeanour in His presence to be rather too familiar but despite more than the requisite degree of awe on my part, it cannot be helped; God is my friend. He was already living in our house when I was born and, undoubtedly blessed with the patience of Job, a phenomenal capacity for forgiveness and a notable sense of humour, He has continued to remain in residence ever since. Until I was about ten years old, in fact, I thought everyone was in on the wonderful, invisible secret, the key to the magical world 'without' and a friend for the mystical world 'within'. Up until we each turned sixteen, church attendance was a non-negotiable part of our week. Though, at a certain point, my motivation to comply admittedly strayed from a passion for Biblical stories to a passion for choirboys, my enthusiasm remained more or less constant. However, although church and Sunday School were undoubtedly bound up with the 'secret', somehow they were not more so than everything else in my day-to-day life. Whilst my gradual discovery that even my father, in the best possible way an exceptional role-model in terms of 'Christian' values, struggled to relinquish himself to the ultimate suspension of disbelief, may, from my early teens, have led me to question the more 'official' faces of religion, happily it did little to sway my deep-down consciousness of God as a part of who I am.

It was not, then, within the hallowed walls of our ancient church that I sought communion with Him but rather, as I had done since a little child, in the miraculous world around me; the trees, the sky, the fields; through observation of the tiniest of insects or that moment when a tight-furled bud yields to the soft, new-green of its leafy charge. Sometimes when I feel the wind on my face I know that God is speaking to me: His reassurance comes not in words but still He is reminding me that He is, and will always be, there.

Deep-down I hear Him.

This hotline to the heavens has carried me through a lifetime of uncertainties, fears, joys and decision-making and I knew it wouldn't let me down now. Nevertheless, there had been occasion as a child for me to accept that, whilst God was ALWAYS listening, I could not expect to be at the front of the, doubtless extremely long, queue every time. Miracles don't always happen overnight. Well this time I could only hope that He was as aware as I was that time was most definitely of the essence; whilst Mrs C. was fantastically understanding about my position, she had made it very clear that the more swift my decision, the less the disruption upon the family, and I had determined to respect that. From a more selfish point of view the whole indecision thing was, as they say, 'doing my head in'. I had to know where I was going…
"Dear God, help me to find the wisdom to choose well", I prayed. "Send me a sign, something to show me which way is the right way – and, P.S., please let the small pimple right on the end of my nose disappear in time for the party tomorrow evening. Thank you."

It is important here to stress that my role immediately following such an appeal is rather more 'pro-active' than one might, at first thought, surmise. Far from resting upon my laurels and waiting upon an imminent flash of lightning to illuminate my path, there follows a time of intense personal and external reflection in the hope of actually recognising the sign when it arrives. There could be nothing more frustrating than suspecting that the answer had been right under one's nose only for its arrival to have coincided with the moment that one had been idly Saving the Universe whilst upside-down and thus for it to be lost forever somewhere in the ether. Still more concerning, it might, for lack of its true target, mistakenly re-appear as the timely, if nonsensical, answer to someone else's eternal conundrum.

(Plus it can't hurt to use the spot cream too. Belt and braces and all that.)

When The Bolt came, once again it was down the telephone. Who'd have thought that God was such a fan of the old blower? For the past five years I'd had nothing but stick from the parental department over my attachment to our home handset and now here it was, God's very own implement of choice! ("OK, admittedly, no… it isn't Himself who pays the bill…")
Anyway, bills aside, my parents were very keen to talk.

Ever since I could remember, there had been a rarely spoken understanding that after school came Oxbridge. My father was a Cambridge man and I had grown up with the golden-hued tales of hallowed halls and punting – not to mention impossibly romantic vignettes of illicit, cloistered visits from my mother. As my passion for learning increasingly bore fruit, so the dreams took on a kind of misty reality – it was just a matter of biding my time. The attendance of two of my brothers at boarding school in Oxford brought still more 'dreaming spires' onto the horizon and often, as I sat with my parents in Christ Church or New College chapel for Sunday evensong, my mind would see me retiring to my own hallowed halls at the end of the service, rather than clambering into the car for the journey home…

At what point things had begun to veer off course it is hard to say exactly but there is no doubt that the bright lights of stage and screen had more than a little to do with enticing me off-route. Music, dance, performance, that exquisite terror in the moment before curtain-up; these became my addiction, fuelled, as they were, by the glorious confidence of youth, brash and raw, as yet undiminished by the wisdom and insecurities of adulthood. Not particularly stretched academically at school and with my own self-discipline curbed by my all-absorbing passion, I slipped increasingly into a relaxed pattern of just doing enough to 'get by'. Where before it had been 'learning' which gave me 'my kicks', in drama and singing I had discovered a whole new and wondrous form of gratification, one of colour, life, music and imagination; a heady combination…

Suffice to say my exam results took a knocking and the Sixth Form saw me at a different school, this time one which prided itself on academic focus. I, accordingly, prided myself in breaking the mould and by the Spring term I was once again my all-singing, all-dancing self, merrily sacrificing 'academic focus' for the thrill of the lights. Though at least here I had competition academically and my naturally competitive streak kept me pretty much afloat, it was, in retrospect, not altogether surprising when the school turned down the irresistible opportunity to prime me for Oxbridge. Ordinarily their faith in my future as being on the stage might have been gratifying, instead I saw it only as a frustrating obstacle to a lifelong dream. Hence Leicester, indecision AND the phone call….

"Well," God said, "what do you think of this for a sign?" I listened. The music swelled. Then, as the words "Oxford" and "interview" broke through the heavenly strains I knew that I had found the 'passion' once again. My heart thumped as my mother took the phone. Oxford were prepared to interview me on the strength of my English grade and some of my written work that my darling, wonderful parents had taken it upon themselves to submit. (Memo; next work should be entitled 'Ghost Writers; a celebration thereof.') If I was happy about it the interview was scheduled for December. Happy??! Happy??! I was delirious. And then terrified. And then delirious. And then terrified all over again. 'Signs' sure are wearing on the nerves.

The warm pricking of tears clouded my eyes and for the first time I realised that for me this wasn't just about Oxford. Once again I was to recall that momentary glimpse of Arabella in the library, head bowed in learning, and I knew that it was indeed about passion, a passion that had been a part of me from the beginning. A passion to see, to learn, to understand; to celebrate the far reaches of the mind and intellect, the power of informed imagination… As the excitement and wonder of discovery flooded through me anew I knew that this time I wasn't going to let it go…

The following days were a whirl. Mrs C. was once again fantastic, countering my concern about letting her down with all kinds of reassuring clichés, along the general lines of 'owing it to myself' and 'taking life by the horns' - or the bull, or something... Anyway suffice to say that she released me from my pact with no hard feelings, which made the whole thing a jolly sight less of a wrench than it might have been. But a wrench, nonetheless, it was. Who would have thought that after only a few months I would have formed such an attachment to my little, (far less homicidal than first suspected), charges? Never had I had such stimulating intellectual debates on Life, The Universe and Everything than with Patch at ten o'clock at night when the Bogeyman was making his evening rounds. My legs were already beginning to feel a cold draught behind the knees in mourning for Tory's little warm body that would no longer share its lovingly restrictive grip whilst queuing for new-warm bread each morning. Who would I find to dance around the garden in a pink bikini with me when Caroline, Marblehead's celebrated striptease artist, was no longer at my side? And baby Katherine…how strange and unexpected the maternal bond that grew with each passing day as I fed, changed and rocked her to sleep in my arms. ..

But there were things to do, planes to book and cases to pack – oh to be a minimalist traveller - friends to hug and old haunts to visit for one last time…

One day I knew I would be back but I knew too, as I looked out over the ocean, that the liquid-gold sun that slid down behind the waves would never again look just as it did now; my spirit, as I climbed the grassy bank above the harbour or skipped along to the now-familiar dunes beyond, would never dance to the same free, unfettered music as it did here and now: And, somewhere inside, I knew too that the tears as I said my quiet farewells were not only for the sea, sky and sun-warmed sands but for the little-girl-woman who was poised just for this moment on the brink of two worlds - and who could never go back…

Chapter Four Reprise
Initiation continued......

It seemed that my condition, which their rigorous tests had confirmed conclusively to be Acute Lymphoblastic Leukaemia (ALL), was by its nature, really a childhood disease. Since the blood was most vulnerable to this specific aberration at a point of development usually characteristic of children under the age of seven, my contracting it at nineteen made me extremely rare. Never one for following the crowd this news might have seen me, (albeit marginally), cheered, were it not for the further revelation that my advanced age, in ALL terms, meant that my chances of survival were significantly reduced. This, combined with the fact that they surmised my body had been battling with the disease, which frequently kills within weeks, if not days, of development, for up to six months, meant that radical action was called for.

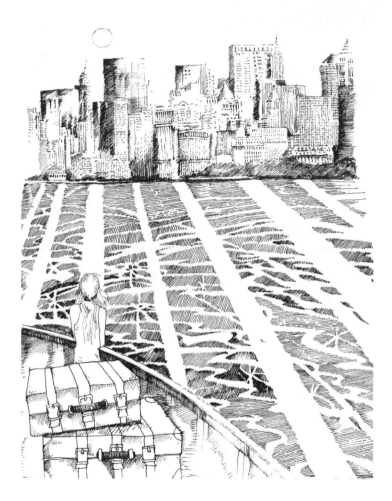

"Out of the blinding light, it rose..."

Chapter Ten

Jessica

My open-return airline ticket simply required a date. Since my flight was from JFK, Mr C. would deposit me - naturally with a good deal of suppressed emotion – at Boston airport in time for the most appropriate internal flight. No problem. Except that the most appropriate internal flight was the day before my GB departure and, touchingly, no-one was prepared for me to risk a night in the Big Apple on my ownsome. Hmmmmm…

And then it came to me. Jessica.

When God was doling out the 'Sugar and Spice' it is quite conceivable that, when it came to my turn, someone jogged his arm. Apart from a couple of enthusiastic tree-climbing years in my early youth I have - for better and worse - always been your quintessential girl's girl. Even diapers and blocked garbage dispensers had duly quaked in the defiant face of pink and blue bikinis, freshly washed hair and discreetly polished nails. However, of all the nannies in our unwittingly exclusive 'club', it was Jessica who really understood the importance of keeping up appearances. The morning wake-up call saw her unfailingly 'enhanced' by a full face of make-up and her stiletto heels were a force to be reckoned with. Whether nine-month-old baby Lauren fully appreciated this morning glory is uncertain but by all accounts her father did and doubtless he was as disappointed as I was when, not long after her arrival, our good-humoured, colourful companion left for the more 'happening' (and hopefully more honourable) state of New Jersey. A down-to earth 'Northern Lass', Jess was warm, direct, honest and great fun to be with and on the strength of a particularly memorable night out at the Boston Hard Rock Café (and a wistful, underage peep through the window of the 'Cheers' bar) she and I had kept in touch. She was, she reported, extremely happy in her new abode. New Jersey had proven itself both in terms of honour and, well, 'happenings' and, positioned on the edge of the water overlooking Manhattan Island, the house was breathtaking. Despite such recommendation and numerous warm invitations by her new host family, I had not as yet had the opportunity to visit but I did recall Jess saying that the Island – and thus by deduction the airport - was but a hop, skip and a private 'ferry'/motorboat-ride from their doorstep. HMMMMMM…!

I rummaged excitedly for my address book and, as God smiled his approval at my train of thought, I knew that this was all part of the plan.

And so, on a warm, bright September morning, with a sky so blue that it almost hurt one's eyes to look at it, the wind whipping my hair and the cool spray teasing my sun-blushed skin, I, and my industrial-sized suitcases, set off for home. As I turned to wave back at Jessica, the motorboat hopping and dancing over the gentle crests, my life panned into wide-screen and I saw us both, small but significant, from above; our smiles and then the sea, the sky, the sleek, modern condos, and, illuminating all, the bright, bright light. And then there was the Island… Out of the blinding light it rose, a mythical, futuristic vision, triumphant and glorious. Manhattan Island, an unashamed celebration of man and his might.

As the camera and I zoomed in, so the awesome two-dimensional skyline took on depth and with it a glimmer of reality. As the bright, heavenly light gave way to the myriad of darks and lights, tones and shadows of a working city, its vast, mystical gates swung open and beckoned me to the life within.

Unperturbed by the weight of my luggage and the lightness of my purse – the sum of my resources (yes, sad-to-say, my university fund) was somewhere in the region of $8 – I sprung out on to the dock, my cases following me in a somewhat less sprightly manner courtesy of the strong-armed ferryman. Momentarily lonesome as I watched the last familiar face pull away, I checked my spirits and set about co-ordinating the next leg of my adventure, which in any event would undoubtedly require a taxi-cab.

Now taxi-cabs, as every good cinema-goer knows, are everywhere in New York City. Well I guess you have heard about that exception that proves the rule - unfortunately, this particular dock seemed to be it. After an optimistic half hour I had to acknowledge that a cab did not seem to be coming to me and on my one valiant attempt to go in search of one I was forced to conclude that Mohammed had undoubtedly packed more sensibly than I had before seeking out that mountain. Then, Halleluja! Just as my loyalties were wearing thin and I was sorely tempted to abandon my worldly goods to their fate and strike out on my own, God's own yellow-cab arrived.

"Hop in!" I sensed Him beam. "And not another thought about those handsome suitcases. They'll be in the back before you can say, 'triple hernia'. Where to now? -As if I didn't know…"

And thus, with a nod to His driver, He left on another call and we were off, in the direction of MOMA, New York's premier museum of modern art.

I was keen to see as much of New York's staggering art heritage as was possible in the short time I had and by all accounts MOMA was the place to start. Too ironically to let pass, (my father would never forgive me!),it is to my own Momma that I owe my continuing passion for art. Her extraordinarily bold decision – yes some said barmy - to take on an Open University Arts degree whilst simultaneously managing the lives of five small children – not to mention my father – not only enriched her appreciation of the inextricable relationship between art, music, literature and life but was to open up my imagination to a whole new world. Peaceful moments curled up with my mother were very often in the prestigious company of the likes of John Everett Millais, JMW Turner, John Ruskin or Jan Vermeer and together we explored their pictorial legacies, the extraordinary language of art tantalisingly revealed to me as she shared the wisdoms of that day's study. A father in publishing and, subsequently, with his own bookshop in Dunstable facilitated a glorious library of prints and books - which inevitably, and disgracefully, has been taken utterly for granted by us all – through which my passion was fed and nurtured. My time at the Gloucestershire gallery finally confirmed my determination to make art my career as well as my love. I had, then, a lot to see and still more to learn and I was impatient to begin…

As we pulled up then outside the museum I hung eagerly out of the window to catch my first glimpse. The fiercely modern façade gave little away about the riches within. 'Riches', yikes! The cab driver had turned and smiled his announcement of our arrival and I suddenly had a reality check. Was it perhaps the case that in this surreal, exotic world, just like at home, one actually had to exchange money for services rendered?!! And, if so, was our journey, during which my driver had had opportunity to hear pretty much my entire life story to date, likely to total less than $8? I thought not. Still, I swung my legs out of the car and, mentally calculating how many times I might need to wash his cab for him in order to pay my dues (at $1 a time?), I put on my most confident smile.

"So, what do I owe you?"

"Well ma'am", he replied, as he tossed the baggage onto the sidewalk as if 'twere mere lettuce leaves; "the deal is that if you go out there and have one hell of a day in our fine city this one's on me."

He grinned, winked, and disappeared and, from somewhere far above, I could swear I heard God chuckle.

Chapter Four Reprise
Initiation continued.....

I would, they informed us, be placed on a trial. Since time was of the essence the dosages of the already highly toxic drugs on the regimen would be doubled in a kind of kill-or-cure attempt to rout the enemy army.

We would have agreed to anything. The world had spiralled out of control, leaving us, dizzy and breathless, clinging desperately to whatever happened to float by. The fact that one of those who did so, Dr O'Hara, had, earlier in her career, worked alongside my Aunt Jane, Mummy's sister, was reassuring. From the outset I knew that her compassion for my condition went beyond the call of duty. She would, I was sure, do everything in her power to defy those odds, and with warmth and humanity.

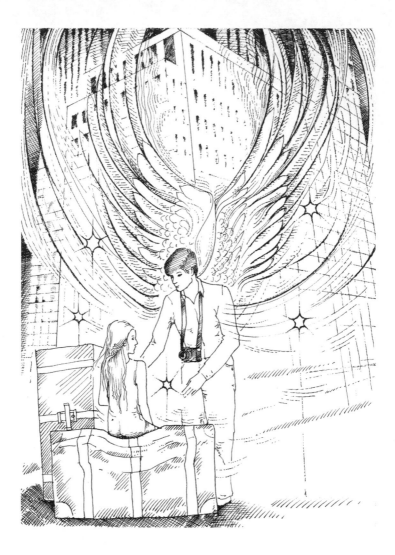

"Excuse me, ma'am" he said angelically.

Chapter Eleven
New York, New York

Now, at the time I was sure that my day in New York was touched by God. From this perspective I can see that it was, in fact, positively escorted by Him; accompanied, no less, by the serenading of angels. Harps and all. Here's why.

God's cab-driver having spirited off whence he came, I looked excitedly across the road at my next point of call. And then down at my cases; and then across; and then down. Sensing the impending risk of a repetitive 'loop' I snapped out of my train of thought. But you can see where I was going. My free-flowing cruise around the museum was sorely in jeopardy but of more immediate concern was the realisation that should I even manage to cross the street, luggage in tow, within the next 24 hours, I would be the exponent of a minor miracle. Hmmmm…?

This time God was more on the ball. Out of the Public Library just behind me stepped a very presentable young man/ angel.

"Excuse me ma'am," he said angelically. "I couldn't help noticing your dilemma. Can I help you with your luggage?"

Resisting the temptation to reply, through gritted teeth, in the affirmative – if, that is, he was in possession of a match and a substantial pyre of wood – I merely smiled gratefully and outlined my plan of action. The fact that the museum had not yet opened for the day – so much for the early bird catching the worm – was, it seemed, to provide a temporary hitch in the proceedings but, he assured me, if I was happy to wait in the early-morning sunshine for half and hour or so he would finish his work in the library and return to help out. I was. And so he did. And, as we chatted 20mins or so later, it transpired that a friend of his was quite high up in the museum and would be delighted, he was sure, to waive the admittance fee for me in the spirit of my adventure. 'Admittance fee?!'. Who'd have thought it? Again my $8 breathed a sigh of relief and an angel carried me over the threshold into the museum.

Naturally with angels in charge even impossibly gi-normous suitcases are swiftly dealt with. His friend was quite happy to look after them at the museum for the day to allow me to explore the city entirely unencumbered!

The angel, it transpired, was actually a photographer, based in Manhattan. There was, he asserted, no other way to see the city in a day than with a true New Yorker. If I would allow it, after my exploration of the museum, he would like to show me the real sights and sounds of The Big Apple, culminating, no less, in an escorted service to the airport. Liberated, excitable, naive, trusting or just plain grateful, I accepted the offer and as the day unfolded it was into one of wonders. In a bright and colourful whirl of new experience, we hit the sights - New Yorker-style: Broadway, Central Park, Chinatown…

As I climbed the steps of my plane home that evening, the last of the day's sun still nurturing the memory of its former glory, it was with a light heart, heavy purse ($8 and 5 cents exactly!), and an internal kaleidoscope of images and impressions, ever changing and modifying through their sleepy filter.

A few minutes later, cocooned in the snug embrace of

seat no.14a, a soft smile still playing dreamily on my lips, my eyelids finally gave in to the temptations of sleep. Carrying me there and across the ocean to the ones I love were the words on the little slip of paper nestling inside my Chinese Fortune Cookie at the end of lunch;

'Of the Lucky, You are the Chosen One...'.

And so I was.

Chapter Four Reprise
Initiation continued.....

Nevertheless, for my parents I could only imagine the anguish. Their ashen but determinedly smiling faces as they arrived each day to take up their vigil by my side belied their own descent into a nightmare realm where no amount of love or force could wrest their child from the capricious hands of fate. Further explanation of the road ahead did little to allay their darkest fears.

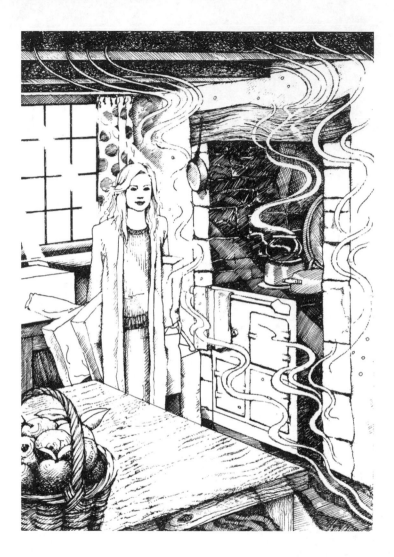

"...how long it seemed since I had stood in our rambling old kitchen and said goodbye."

Chapter Twelve
No place like home

My first sight of Daddy after three long months was a fleeting one. And then another. And another. Each time the security doors swept open his face took on a momentary flash of hope, only to relapse into an increasing expression of concern as the person skipping through them transpired once again not to be me. The fact that the number of male, uniformed companions beside me seemed to be multiplying at a rather alarming rate did little, I imagine, to assuage his unease. To tell you the truth it wasn't doing much to assuage mine either.

Initially I had felt only sympathy for the poor misguided fellow who had so rashly claimed his right to search my luggage. Was he short of things to do over the next three weeks?? Clearly he had bitten off sizeably more than he could chew. Still, thoroughly confident that I had absolutely nothing to declare, I was able to feel virtuously patient at the unnecessary procedure, chirpily answering in the negative each probing question as it arose; drugs, alcohol, cigarettes? I was even rather flattered at his particular interest in the rather snazzy cowboy boots that I had seen instantly would prove an indispensable contribution to my university trousseau. (How pleased Daddy would be!).

"Did you purchase these in the States," the uniform inquired courteously. And then, in response to my cheerful reply in the affirmative, "And anything else? – Clothing; gifts?"

Strangely, as I listed with excitement all the surprise

presents that I had had such fun in choosing over the past few weeks, he seemed far more interested in how much they had cost than the colour, cut or flavour of the respective items. So much so in fact that he seemed to be totting things up with an extraordinary attention to detail as I spoke.

With a final, pointed click of the keyboard he looked up and, in his most officious voice declared;

"There will be £57-50 tax to pay on these goods before we can release you."

I opened my eyes wide. "I do have $8," I said hopefully…

"Where would one be without unconditional love?" I thought contentedly, as I snuggled happily under Daddy's arm on the way to the car. In my case the answer undoubtedly lay in a very uncomfortable place with stern faced officials and harsh bright lights. Instead, released from captivity, cowboy boots and all, I was going home, safe in the knowledge that, to my father at least, it was worth paying to have me back.

Doubtless Daddy's excitement at the bountiful gifts that I was so looking forward to bestowing was somewhat diminished by the knowledge that he had in part footed the bill himself but otherwise he seemed as pleased to see me as I was him. Skipping along beside him, stories and news tumbling out in my joy at sharing my experiences of the past few months, made me acutely aware of how much I had missed everyone and how long it seemed since I had stood in our rambling old kitchen and said goodbye.

Standing once again in the kitchen, the warmth of the big red Aga curling around my travel-worn limbs in a welcoming caress, that day seemed even more distant. How strange everything was. How small the room had become and how low the ancient beamed ceilings. But there was Mummy, smiling from her familiar chair as I ran over to embrace her as though I had been away at least as long as Gulliver. Perhaps, like me, on his return, he too had been struck by the sudden realisation that, whilst his life had been changing irreparably and forever, the world he left behind had carried on just as before.

Here, the early September sun that fingered through the little wood beyond the house had conceded the bright white light of Summer to the rich golden hue of Autumn days. The leaves were beginning to turn and the pleasantly acrid smell of burnt stubble hung in the air. One by one my siblings appeared, first their footsteps sounding on the worn terracotta tiles of the corridor as I took a guess as to whom they belonged. As I spread out the gifts on the big farmhouse table, a wizened apple in one hand, stolen as of old from the motley selection in the large basket, I knew I was truly home.

It was only as that first wave of excitement and newness had passed that I realised just how exhausted I was. The overwhelming need to sleep washed over me in an all-consuming tide and it was all I could do to stumble up the little back stairs to my so familiar/so strange bedroom and fall between the cool sheets. Not even the imminent arrival of my boyfriend, Ben, could hold sway over the all-powerful dominion of sleep...

Chapter Four Reprise
Initiation continued......

As we understood it, the first year would see me almost entirely in hospital. Here my already disease-ravaged body would be subjected to an intensive combination of cytotoxic (or 'chemo') drug and radio-therapy in the hope of holding back the most imminent danger. Assuming it were possible for me to attain remission, I would then follow a two year maintenance course of oral and intravenous drugs in an attempt to consolidate the effect of those initial months. Even if I made it that far, there were no guarantees that my newly established system would not collapse once the drugs were withdrawn. And after that…well, only time would tell.

Chapter Thirteen
Crossroads

My mother will be the first to confirm that after the initial rosy period of reuniting and rediscovery came the Dark Ages. Long days where she and I suffered in equal amounts the down-side of my new-found independence. My frustrations at finding myself no longer at liberty to plan my own time or to roam at will beyond the confines of home and, above all, at my lack of focus now that I had abandoned one course and still had yet to strike out upon another were rendering me intolerable to live with. Naturally I was less willing to acknowledge this at the time than at this safe distance, and thus my poor parents took the blame. Thankfully for all concerned there was hope on the horizon. There was the Oxford interview to finalise, the good old gallery in Glos. and new excitement at the possibility of my attending a six month art history course in Florence. At this point in time, I suspected, nowhere could be too far where my mother was concerned but, content to see the latter plan perhaps take fruit in early January, she helped me to pack in the meantime for good old Gloucestershire and the home of Kate, one of her oldest and dearest friends and the manageress of the Kenulf gallery.

My weeks there earlier in the summer had been idyllic. My memory is as a patchwork of colours. The subtle, age-softened hues of 19th century paint; the deep red of the lunchtime tomatoes; the clotted-cream yellow of Cotswold stone in the late afternoon light; the mystery of greens that were the wooded hillside beyond the house where Kate and I roamed in search of glow-worms and the new-white spines of Henry the baby hedgehog that we rescued and brought up as our own. How on the brink of everything I was and how eager to look and learn and remember.

For me, to return was to have never been away. This time too there was London. The first art fairs of the season had begun and I relished the contrast between sleepy Winchcombe and the bustle and glamour of the vast capital. Here the very fabric of the city exuded possibility; the walls whispered of dreams and visions, past, present and future. Deep down I determined that I too would be a part of that history, that, one day, the walls would tell of my world, of my dreams, and perhaps draw another young dreamer a little closer to her goal.

Thus inspired and with the knowledge that the Kenulf's permanent London venture was still very much 'in progress', the final week of my time in the city saw me pushing open the chic, glass door to Chelsea's 'Wilson and Gough Gallery' in bold response to their advertisement for a new recruit. With the relaxed, happy confidence that can only truly be the province of the blissfully naive, I smiled and chatted my way through the interview, my genuine enthusiasm for the role and its creative, cutting edge environment shining in my eyes. Five days later I was back. This time I had my own desk.

How strange and exhilarating is the path of fate. How strong and purposeful the hand that guides. As the days passed, the mighty city unveiled itself before me, shedding its evening cloak of glamour in humble, tacit acknowledgement of my new 'belonging'. The sight and sounds of early morning London; the rumble, clank, hiss of the refuse vans as they devour the remains of yesterday in preparation for the arrival of today; the slippery, putrid cabbage leaf that still clings to the Chelsea pavement, its former glory usurped by the gleaming array of new produce that shouts ostentatiously 'Red, Green, Orange, Yellow', from the safety of its shop front stalls; the dusky-faced youths with their antiquated dust-carts, dark eyes to carry one to far-away exotic places; the cat-calling builders grinning in doorways, celebrating the late arrival of the foreman; the thin, spare form, ever-shrinking beneath his pile of filthy rags, pleading for 'any spare change' before he is once again moved on and the wizened bag-lady who forages for hidden treasures in the Park Lane bins; these were features of the hidden face, behind the showman's mask, without which the show could not go on.

Finally came the actors. With a mighty heaving from the city's underbelly, the Tube, far beneath the well-worn pavements, came the cast, right on cue: a slick, chic tide spewing onto the streets; spreading and dispersing outwards from their underground source towards singular pre-programmed destinations; a perfumed, coiffed and pinstriped army, indomitable in its purpose, absolute in its infiltration. Technically, of course, I too was part of this army and deep-down revelled in my inclusion in this new, powerful force. In part though I remained the observer, determined, as I was, never to become just one more ghost in the machine. Thus, even as my own heels click-clicked their way towards their goal, my film camera was rolling from above, now 'panning in' and now 'wide-focus', telling and re-telling the daily story.

Eight hours after, (and just as surely as), its initial onslaught, the army retreated. As the film span into rewind mode so the tide gathered volume and momentum; the trickle of innumerable, lonely rivulets converging to re-form that almighty flood upon which they would once again sail out whence they came.

Tired but elated, I too was swept up in the nightly exodus,

the Express coach weaving its way through the evening lights towards home. And each night, just for a moment, as I pressed my nose against the glass pane beside me, I was a child again, looking out upon a twinkling wonderland...

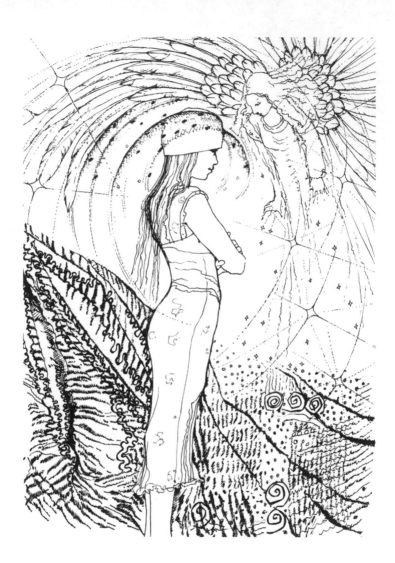

"Whether this actually meant 'try on all the hats', is admittedly debatable..."

Chapter Fourteen
Potholes

Those first few days became a week, then two and then three. How quickly I adjusted to my dual world; by day a fledgling butterfly, learning how to spread my wings in the glittery garden of SW3; as darkness fell, flitting tirelessly as a moth, in my familiar home-world with family, friends and the ever-patient Ben.

Except that I wasn't really tireless but, truth be known, increasingly exhausted by my bid to maintain both lives to the fullest, carried for now on the duplicitous wings of adrenalin. Ben, too, was becoming less and less patient in terms of my commitment to the future. My coming home meant facing up to the realities of my new-found independence – being in control of my own life was not all about freedom from restraints but primarily about managing the responsibilities I had, not only to myself but also to those around me, in the most wise and positive way possible. Where Ben was concerned I was aware that the day-by-day basis on which I had approached our teenage relationship hitherto, (not so much casual – it was loving and committed – but rather without a thought for where we might be going long-term), was no longer adequate. New, 'grown-up' issues were raising their head, 'birth-control', it seemed, shouting the loudest and most persistently. Decisions that, from beyond the sea, I had banked on having an entire year to form were confronting me hard and fast and I was increasingly aware of feeling less and less equipped to make them. My candle was being well and truly burnt from both ends but life was new and exciting and each night as I shed my butterfly wings and assumed my nocturnal guise I put aside such cares and celebrated being alive.

Needless to say my mother's fear that I was pushing too hard fell, at least for a time, on deaf ears. As if I didn't have enough to contend with without her ongoing insistence that I see a doctor to alleviate her concerns! Three weeks into a new job, I insisted equally firmly, was not the ideal stage at which to request time out. Finally, however, maternal love (and persistence) won out. I had admittedly been deficient in iron at various points since aged 12 or 13 and if a two-minute consultation with our doctor resulting in a prescription for iron tablets would ease her mind then go I would.

Easier said than done! Getting past the battleaxes on the reception desk (we are convinced there must be a special qualification required for the post) was nothing short of a Herculean task. They had 'absolutely nothing' for nearly three weeks and even then it was with the extremely dubious doctor who, on more than one occasion, had well and truly leapt over the line where ethical behaviour was concerned. Mummy was not impressed. When crossed she takes on more than a passing resemblance to my grandmother who has in her time had many a grown 'official' quaking in his brogues. We call this phenomenon 'doing the scary Mummy'. Best not to be around when it is going on. Anyway, suffice to say, 'scary Mummy' did the trick and miraculously a hole had appeared in the schedule for two days time.

The waters in the meantime smooth once again, I buzzed thankfully back to the Big Smoke, where my new boss was far more understanding than I was about the impending hiatus. I spent a rather blissful day wandering around the Chelsea Crafts Fair, which, I discovered, far from comprising, as I had suspected, numerous unidentifiable objects made from wicker and the odd 'corn dolly' (what on earth are these actually for?), was an altogether more sophisticated affair. To a Londoner, 'craft' seemed to comprise primarily of exquisite items of jewellery, clothing and more hats,(my particular weakness), than you could shake a stick at and, if this was not cool enough, I was being paid by the hour to investigate thoroughly. Whether this actually meant 'try on all the hats', is, admittedly, debatable but I have never been one to leave a stone unturned… Anyway, needless to say, at the end of my assignment, I arrived back at the gallery with a broad smile and a spring in my step.

Mummy's phone call then was a particular shock. The very fact that she was calling me at work rang my alarm bells but I was not prepared for her shaky voice. My father, it seemed, had had a car accident on the hairy early-morning run to deliver my brother to the school coach. Taking a bend too fast, his Mercedes had slammed into a lamppost, catapulting him and Jeremy and William out of their seats. The car was utterly written off but by some miracle all three had escaped with whiplash and 'minor injuries'. We had oft joked about the lethal 6.45am race to beat the clock (and I must say the odds, given that the party always left a good four minutes later than the absolute latest) – it would be a joke no longer.

My heart had stood still as she relayed the news. Now I found that I too was trembling with a mixture of relief and the initial shock. For all of our family, I knew, this event would have a lasting impact. It was as if we had hitherto been surrounded by a golden bubble; a protective shield that ensured that the 'sticks and stones' that life threw out merely bounced off. Life behind our high red-brick wall was one of sunshine, tangled flowers and home-made strawberry milkshake and this simply didn't fit. Only the extraordinary fortune that had saved the accident from being more serious would save us from losing entirely our perhaps naive but oh so important trust in life.

Instinctively I wanted to be at home, holding on to my family for dear life, squeezing everlasting security into them with the force of my love. A more rational voice, however, asserted, as had my mother, that, given that the immediate drama was over, to finish my day's work would be the responsible thing, and I consoled myself in the knowledge that due to the pesky doctor's appointment I would be safely back in the nest the following day...

Chapter Fifteen
Drama Queen

I was, frankly, reluctant to go anywhere the following day, let alone to face the demon receptionists who would doubtless be mumbling things about preferential treatment, 'scary Mummys' and the like, but a deal was a deal and at least it meant I had the rest of the day at home. So, with the only bus that passed through our one-horse village fortunately going in the right direction, 9.30am saw me sitting patiently in the surgery waiting room, with only a few well-worn copies of Readers Digest for company. The following hour in said seat gave me plenty of time to dwell upon two notable phenomena; firstly, (quite baffling), that the magazines appeared, by way of their condition, to have been of such profound interest to so many, and secondly, (still more disconcerting), the fact that despite my interminable sojourn in the 'waiting room' – how aptly named – being such a solitary one, a whole surgery full of doctors was clearly, and at great length, up to their eyes in something behind those eerily closed doors. I was just beginning to realise that these two phenomena were inextricably linked and with it lose my nerve altogether when my name crackled over the tannoy system.

Dr Kilpatrick is as reassuring a fellow as you are ever likely to meet. His presence shouts 'Doctor', in the storybook sense, every bit as loudly as does his big, battered, brown leather bag. When he reaches over to grab his stethoscope I find myself anticipating the Fischer Price version - splendid in all its primary colours – every time. But no; he is also a real doctor and the needle that he inserted as sensitively as possible into my arm was undoubtedly a real needle. Ouch!

Commenting that I did look a little pale, he assured me that the results of my blood test would be back in a couple of weeks and that perhaps I should take things a little more slowly for a while until my system had picked up. With more than a slight suspicion that he was well and truly in cahoots with another interested party and wondering how I had missed the additional side-effect of burning ears a couple of days earlier, I left the surgery with a slightly sore arm, a small sticking plaster and a smiley, warm feeling that was a symptom of someone who realises they are very well loved indeed...

Given his estimated time lapse of two weeks, I was quite surprised to answer the telephone to Dr K. that very afternoon. The hospital, he said, were keen to confirm the results of my test the following morning – would I be available to call in at 10am?

Would I?! How cool was that?! All the way through school I had been sickeningly healthy. As friends all around me were fainting in assembly, having allergic reactions to chocolate (this one did at least benefit me directly, especially around Easter time) and all manner of exciting things, I remained stoically well, the drama queen in me only able to look enviously on as said heroines were carried limply to the waiting car... Besides one or two suspected fractures I had only ever set foot in a hospital when Mummy was having another baby – granted this had made me quite a regular – but it wasn't quite the same as having one's own flowers and jugs of weak orange squash. Who knew – they might even let me stay in! Tripping merrily down the stairs and into the kitchen I let Mummy know the exciting news.

Seeming rather less enamoured of the idea than I was,

she immediately mumbled something about calling Will's headmaster to rearrange a meeting and dashed off into the library. After collecting a drink for myself, I dashed off after her, keen, on the realisation that I didn't have a thing to wear, to get a bid in for her new negligee, an extremely pretty, extremely minimal and extremely optimistic gift from my father, just in case I was allowed to stay. As I pushed open the door the force of my reception was not unlike that faced by fireman in the heat of a blaze – I believe it is known as 'backdraft'.

"Get out, get out, get out!" Mummy yelled at me from the 'telephone chair' as I staggered backwards out of the room. Poor Will. Clearly he had this time done something that really was beyond the pale… 'Scary Mummys' are best left to themselves. The nightdress would just have to wait…

That night as I dressed for dinner – Ben and I were meeting up with his brother and his girlfriend and a few other friends for a birthday celebration at a nearby restaurant – Mummy came up the little steps into my room and sat down on the bed. Her eyes shining with love she looked across at me in the warm red lamplight, (I was in my surreal lighting phase), and smiled gently.

"Why don't you stay here tonight," she suggested quietly. "I won't go out and we could have a peaceful evening together with a book and some music."

I smiled too and picked up my belt from its strategic position on the sofa. "How about tomorrow, Mummy?" I replied cheerily. "Oh, listen, that must be my lift! See you later!" And I flitted off into the night…

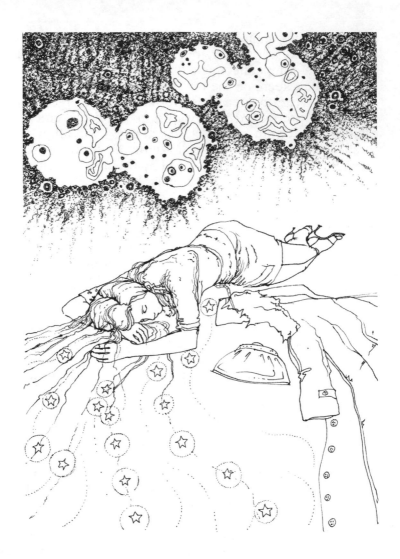

"And I collapsed on the carpet."

Chapter Sixteen
Signpost

I didn't give my forthcoming adventure another thought until right at the end of the meal. Amidst the laughing and joking Ben explained that we wouldn't be able to meet up with the others the following day after all. "Off to Oxford already are we?" Alex ribbed. "No," Ben replied quietly, "she has to go in to hospital."

A hush fell across the room. Suddenly it didn't seem quite like the jolly jaunt that I had been anticipating. I smiled cheerfully. "There's no drama," I insisted, "I doubt they'll even let me stay in." A mumbled chorus of 'rather you than me's' and the like signalled the start of normal banter once again and Ben and I caught eyes across the table. A sudden chill ran through me and I touched my feet against his for reassurance. "Ben, what if it's leukaemia?" I whispered, barely audibly. Without words he reached over and took my hand.

Then, with the intricate business of 'bill division' well and truly taken care of, the evening signalled its end. Coats were summoned, farewells called.

And I collapsed on the carpet.

I remember little about the journey home, save being carried (heroine-like!) to the car. And at least it wasn't an allergy to chocolate...

Chapter Seventeen
Guidance

The next morning dawned fair and all trace of the previous night's drama had left peacefully on the wings of sleep. Nevertheless I was beginning to acknowledge that perhaps Mummy was right – a few of those iron tablets would not go amiss. I finished packing my small overnight bag – well you never know! – the coveted nightdress folding satisfyingly into a slippery bundle approximately the size of a child's pocket handkerchief. As I bounced downstairs and into the car my head was full of imaginings about the day ahead.

"Do you think they will let me stay, Mummy?" I asked hopefully, leaning over her seat from behind as we drove along. "They might," she replied simply. I sat back contentedly.

Only a slight shadow hung over the proceedings, in the form of 20- odd small pills secreted in the bottom of my bag. My final decision to take the contraceptive pill had by no means been easily reached. For one thing I hated taking such an important step without consulting my mother. She and Daddy had adopted from early on what I feel to be an immensely wise – and brave – policy with regard to our upbringing. Rather than, from the moment we hit our teens, surrounding us with a fortress of ' Do not, must not, cannots, that just cried out to be escaped from, they operated a school of 'advice'. Granted some of the 'advice' was handed out more forcefully than the rest, but in general we felt able to talk to them about most things, reassured by the knowledge that we could then weigh up their adult wisdom before taking the foolhardy plunge that we of course realised was the only way to go. In fact, naturally, sometimes we did decide that we knew best and doubtless it is through such painful learning experiences that one attains wisdom and nirvana. On more than one occasion, though, our respect for mater or pater caused us to think more than twice about our impending decision and, as such, has doubtless saved me, at least, from one or two potentially 'uncomfortable' experiences.

Over this one, though, I agonised long and hard. In the past Mummy had dealt utterly frankly and honestly with me over the issue of sex and, whilst where this particular matter was concerned, sound advice had buckled under the overwhelming torrent of raging hormones, somehow just having confided in my mother - and friend – had lent a stability and maturity to the situation that was invaluable in terms of my emotional well-being. (Though, admittedly, it may not have done much for Mummy's!) Where the pill was concerned I guess it felt like pushing that broad-mindedness just a little too far. My own insecurities about making such a commitment, not only in terms of my relationship but also in embarking on what is essentially a course of drug therapy, doubtless, (ironically), contributed to my reluctance to broach the subject. I have for as long as I can remember been passionately averse to taking any form of drug/medication that is not absolutely necessary. I would rather cope with a bearable headache than take a painkiller; let a cold run its course than stuff myself up further with so-called remedies that merely mask the symptoms that are the body's way of dealing with it naturally. Mummy has always asserted that the reason we were all so healthy in comparison to friends when the cold/cough/flu bugs were raging was good old-fashioned roaming around draughty corridors, enhancing our resilience and building up our immune systems. Though at the time, shivering in our overcoats around the Aga – visitors would arrive (at their peril) only to enquire politely and with faint surprise where we were off to and to be met with the equally surprised, uncomprehending reply of "nowhere" from those for whom the wearing of outdoor clothing indoors had become a mere matter of course – we suspected a hefty dose of propaganda in this, I have to say that I can think of no better explanation. Anyway suffice to say I have a great deal of faith in my body to look after itself provided I look after it and this to my mind meant pills were out. Nevertheless, the combined pressure of the old hormones, both his and mine, and the knowledge, flagged pointedly in my direction by my dear Mamma, that we were as a rule an extremely fertile family, was a daunting opponent and that very week had seen me finally give in.

Now, as my fingers toyed thoughtfully with the little packet, I hoped fervently that the issue would not come up whilst we were with the doctor and before I felt ready to talk to Mummy about things myself.

Then, with a sudden right-hand turn, the subject was closed. Swung well and truly out of my reverie I sat up and looked out along the hospital driveway. We had arrived and, as we bumped over the sleeping policemen into the car park, I wondered what adventures lay around this bend…

Chapter Four Reprise
Initiation complete!!!!

As far as I was concerned, my survival was a given. The real horror resided in the fight that lay ahead. The next few years seemed like an eternity – an endless landscape of pain and fear from which I could surely never emerge as whole.

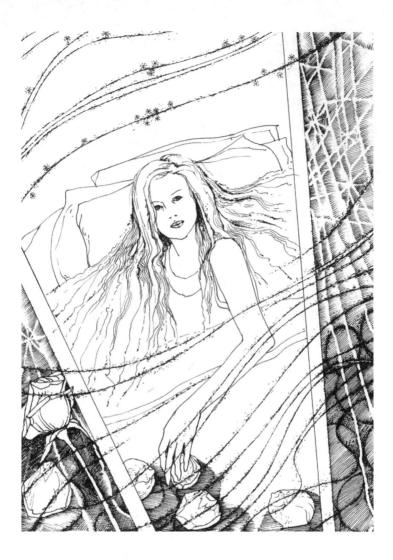

"...as one by one the petals began to fall..."

Chapter Eighteen
The Tide

And then they came. Dozens and dozens of people, filing in past the beady eye of the ward sister, snaking their way down the long white corridors to wait patiently outside my room to be 'received'.

There I lay, 'in state', propped by four plump pillows to greet them one by one, two by two, as they came. Into this strange, surreal world they kept coming, borne on a tide of love and compassion that all but swept me away with the glory and might of its force. My one single life had somehow touched so many. Time and place had been 'condensed', to converge in this tiny room, where nursery friends smiled shyly at boyfriends past and present as they passed in the doorway and A-level teachers exchanged polite greetings with those who had inspired me in my first years at school.

It was, we said, like seeing God; flowing in and out of that ward, reminding us that He was there, that He would never abandon us.

Those first few days, of course, were hardest for those who truly loved me. For my grandparents, perched tearfully beside me on the bed, I knew that in part the grieving for my loss had already begun. Strangely it was I who smiled and comforted, squeezing their hands as if to reassure them of the life still burning within me. For Ben too, I was simply fading away. The single white rose that he lay beside me, as if upon my grave, was me; its life was my life and, as one by one the petals began to fall, so he saw that life ebb irretrievably from my already fragile form. This time we had together he knew to be our last. As he brushed, oh so gently, my long, still shining hair it was, for him, to be the last time; as my hair, like the petals, began to fall, so it would be never to return.

Still, while those around me cried and grieved, there I lay, smiling, touching and affirming from behind my wall. From the other side I watched the real world come in and then go out again; back to the cars, buses and trains, to the parties, interviews and sports games that somewhere inside I recalled having once known - long ago. The November 5th fireworks that spat and crackled far-off in the night sky belonged to a time long past – or perhaps merely to a dream, but sleepily recalled?

And then the tide stopped rolling. Two weeks after I built my wall, the hospital machine took back control; the corridors were silent and the long-ago world took its final leave.

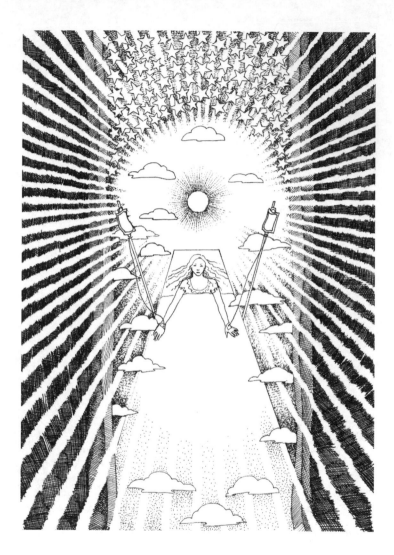

"It was necessary... to isolate me from the outside world."

Chapter Nineteen
Isolation

Much of these early weeks were to be spent in isolation. In effect, I surmised, ALL is a cancer of the immune system. The white, immune cells develop a deformity, whereby they reproduce, in a damaged form, progressively more rapidly, at the expense of the other cells in the blood. The result is not only the systematic destruction of immunity. The increasing lack of red blood cells as a consequence causes the body to become starved of vital oxygen – were it not that dying is usually precipitated by an irresistible infection, the untreated leukaemia victim would slowly suffocate to death. Hmmm. Nice.

In treating the disease, the regimen proposed would seek to destroy utterly those rogue cells in the hope that the body would rally in defence and put forth a new bank of immune cells, minus the 'blip'. Unfortunately the drugs administered were unable to discriminate between healthy and deformed cells, having rather more of the 'bull-in-a-china-shop' approach to the task in hand than I fancied was ideal, and as such my entire immune system would be wiped out. They hoped temporarily.

The hiatus between this initial onslaught and my body's triumphant return to form would be critical. With absolutely no means of defence in the face of infection, even a cold could prove fatal. It was necessary therefore to remove, as far as possible, any potential source of such an infection and thus to isolate me from the outside world. Even the innocent cut flower, it seemed, was a risk, apparently harbouring potentially dangerous bacteria.

Flowers I could survive without. My family was another matter. The doctors had agreed to allow my parents occasional access to my room, but my brothers and sister, with their daily exposure to the inevitable bugs that were doing the school rounds, were strictly off limits.

Those final few days of the 'induction' period then were poignant ones. My family represented for me all that was happy and secure. They were nights spent boldly in garden tents, munching sausage sandwiches; days passed excitedly on seaside piers and long 'healthy walks' in the countryside, bribed by the promise of a hard-won ice-cream at the journey's end. They were bickering and grumbles, loving and laughter – and they were a part of me. How ironic then to be severed from them just at the time when my spirit cried out for them most.

From their perspective too, I imagined, not being able to see me on a regular basis, to smile and tease and know first hand that I was still holding on, would be hard. The darkest fear of all is the unknown; the imagination feeds so greedily on the boundless and the unseen. Selfishly I was glad that if any one of us were to be so dangerously sick, then it was I. To watch one of the others suffering would be anguishing; to be isolated from them in that suffering would be intolerable. I had never been so conscious of the depth of my love for them all. It grew and swelled inside me with a pain that threatened to burst the physical bounds that contained it; I wanted with every ounce of me to show them the strength of that love, for them to know that even whilst we were kept apart it would be there inside me, binding me to them and guiding me through the dark.

That love, the memories of a long-ago place where there was always an answer and the quaking shadows never lost their fear of the light; these would become my reality.

My inner world would be my life; my imagination would people the stark, lonely room – fill its silent walls with the words and laughter that the past 19 years had left resounding in my ears...

Chapter Twenty
The Wall

From the beginning of that third week, all those who did enter my little room were required to wear a decidedly un-becoming range of polythene accessories in what I saw to be a not merely unflattering but also rather ineffectual attempt to protect me from the world without. Still, it was good for a chuckle. The potential humour in the sight of Daddy, shrink-wrapped, was not to be passed up, despite the general air of tragedy about the place – Jeremy would never have forgiven me.

Every morning at 8am, the cheerful, Filipino cleaning lady would breeze in. Suitably attired in a rather fetching green plastic, she bustled about the room sweeping and disinfecting any potential bug into submission whilst I munched Rice Crispies and listened to her tales about her family back home. The breakfast menu was somewhat limited. Indeed the hospital food in general seemed rather to be an exercise in irony than a genuine working proposition for sick people. Almost entirely comprised of the kind of food that falls neatly under the cliché of 'a heart-attack-waiting-to-happen' with the remainder from the Rice Crispie school of 'all air and no substance', the daily fare seemed staggeringly inappropriate. After watching me wade through yet another bowl of steamed pudding and custard, Mummy broke. Her initial fury fired by the discovery that all the meals were delivered daily, (already on their plates – how convenient!), from Newcastle and reheated in the microwave on arrival, she was decided. From then on she would bring me good, home-cooked food each day. Beside my bed was my emergency hamper, a wicker basket of my favourite nonperishable goodies; Marmite, WholeEarth Peanut Butter, home-made muesli and porridge oats for breakfast and impromptu attacks of the munchies. Day after day my amazing mother prepared and delivered exquisite plates of mange-touts, steak and kidney pie, broccoli cheese, her famous egg custard or my grandfather's home-made leek soup, laden with nutrition and love to urge my body on to health. Yummmmm.

And then, all of a sudden, I didn't care any more.

When they had said that some of the drugs – and one in particular, Daunerubenstein - would make me sick, they didn't tell me that my body would be turned inside out; that my mind would warp with the anguish and that for ever after my eyes would carry a deep, dark remembering. Even the sight of the huge syringe with its dark, poisonous-red contents belied the evil that was to follow its slow insidious journey through my unsuspecting veins. As then, and with each subsequent onslaught, the lining of my tummy rent and tore with the force of my retching, I knew that so too the heart of whichever of my parents was there beside me bled in pain. As my body writhed and heaved in agonised desperation to rid itself of this evil invader, I built my wall a few bricks higher and knew that the world had truly lost its senses.

Chapter Twenty One
Hair Today, Gone Tomorrow

The drug regimen, as I came to understand it, consisted firstly of those, like Daunerubenstein, that came under the banner 'chemotherapy', specifically targeted to ALL; Methotrexate, 6Mercaptapurine; Vinchristin; an antibiotic, Co-Trimoxizole and a hefty dose of Prednisolone, or steroids, which would help counteract the damaging effects of the chemo.

My little body needed all the help it could get. Before the curtain came down on the two-week prologue, I had been confronted with a decision: 'To shave or not to shave?' Losing my hair, they said, was, regrettably, inevitable. Although there were in some cases methods to protect the scalp from the effects of chemotherapy, the proposed radiation treatment to my head would ensure that any remaining wisps would be lost anyway. As the drugs began to work their way deeper into my system, so my hair would begin to fall.

The weight of long hair, they explained, tends to pull the hair out more quickly, and generally patients tend to opt for shaving their heads entirely before the whole gruesome process kicks in. Certainly the idea of bare patches of scalp interspersed with the long strands of hair that were still 'hanging in there' was disturbing, a haunting image born of night-time demons. Nevertheless, the idea of shaving my head was absolutely abhorrent. There was, for me, something inherently aggressive, even destructive, in such an action and, with so radical an approach to preempting the hair-loss, a kind of ruthless abandonment of the last vestige of sanity and reality. For a girl in particular, too, I think, her hair is a way of expressing who she is inside. The long, fair hair that still brushed my back when I moved spoke in such different tones to the rough bristles of a shaven scalp. Why are soldiers shorn of their worldly haircut on recruitment, or, I reflected, why were the concentration camp Jews ritually shaven if not, in part, to suppress individual identity? So, I felt, in this way I would be giving myself up entirely to this new dictator, my disease. No, if I were, as I must, to heed their advice then I would do it my way.

As the smiling nurse showed Mummy and Heather into my room that evening, I once again marvelled at the extraordinary power of love and compassion. Heather was my hairdresser and she wanted to help. What she knew was hair, and if there was anything that she could do then she would be right there, scissors in hand.

All of a sudden this was about choice. As she and I, heads bowed, contemplated the ideas page that I had compiled, debating the merits of one short, arty crop versus another, I even began to feel a twinge of excitement about the radical new style. The last time I had tried out the 'short and chic' approach to hair, I was about two years old. Granted, thanks to my mother, I was a proud model of the very latest in asymmetric fringes but I had nevertheless been somewhat wary of revisiting the look ever since.
'Well,' I thought, 'here goes nothing..!'

Amidst much animated chat and giggling, the final decision made, the scissors started to whirr. For an hour or so my strange little room was a bright, happy salon – though naturally with only the most select of clients and with nightwear being the only way to dress, dah..ling!

101

As the long tresses of hair fell to the floor it was with the thrill of daring rather than the pain of loss that I squeezed Mummy's hand.

When Heather finally held the mirror up before me I hardly dared open my tight-shut eyes. Then, from the moment I did, I could not stop peeping at my new, elven self. I loved it and, most importantly, it was another victory to my spirit in the ongoing battle with the unseen enemy.

I did not have long to celebrate victory…

That first morning that I awoke choking on the thousands of tiny strands of hair that filled my nose, mouth and lashes, the nightmare, cackling in triumph, severed entirely my link with the old world.

As for Samson before me, my hair had become my defiance. Whilst it remained, resolutely resisting the threat that flowed daily through my veins, I knew that I was winning. If my hair was not falling out, as it was predicted to do, then it followed that sickness and dying similarly were merely inexplicably cruel threats calculated to test my fighting spirit. If I just held on a little longer, the bell would sound, time would be up and I would go home, proudly purveying my advanced certificate from the 'University of Life'.

Instead, it seemed, I was to be forced to face a new reality, to accept this place of unimaginable fears as my here and now. Well then, like Samson, I was not going to go down without a fight.

And fight I would have to do. As each morning I choked and cried, drowning in the unnatural manifestation of terrors that my mind could not even acknowledge, a small part of me was changed forever. How much hair one has to lose. At first the loss was hardly noticeable, my new chic crop holding its own against the onslaught; but I knew. To touch my hand against my head was to see ever more come away, finally to reveal the delicate pink of the skin beneath. Then there were only tiny wisps left. Fine, baby blond strands of hair that took me back nineteen years to the little girl that no-one could ever have imagined would now be fighting death, before her life had really begun. As my parents stroked my small, naked head I sensed the years rolling backwards, had never before been so aware of being their little girl; who may be all grown up but would always be their baby…

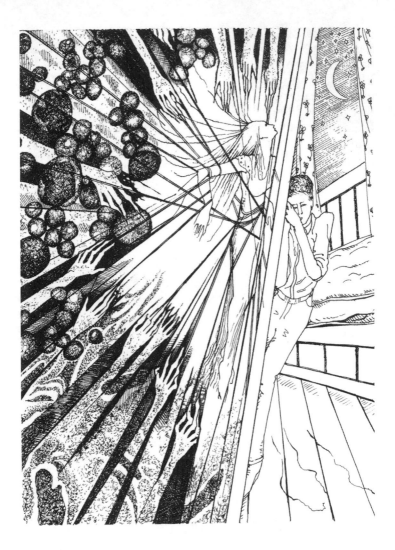

"...warping and distorting our fragile inner world."

Chapter Twenty Two
Demons

For Ben, coming to terms with my unnatural transition from vibrant young woman back to vulnerable child was never going to be easy. The fact that, as he saw it, this was merely the preamble to my inevitable death made it positively tortuous. His hopeless despair was almost tangible, made still more agonising for us both by his sudden swings into absolute denial. With each passing day we could only watch, helpless, as the brick wall between us grew in stature. Alternately we reached out desperately across the divide, young, confused and terrified, only to recoil in horror in finding our ally resolutely cementing the next brick. Each torn up from the root and flung swirling through our own black abyss of fear and isolation, neither of us was equipped to draw the other gently back to earth. Devoid of certainty, security and, in Ben's case, hope, there were no reassuring platitudes to soothe and calm the fevered mind.

I had always been the one he could be real with, the one who knew the vulnerable child behind the tall, strong young man who was invincible, impenetrable and knew no fear. To the outside world I played along happily in the role of damsel to his knight, revelling in the old-fashioned boy-girl ideal of protector and protected. Deep down, though, that very vulnerability that seemed to flutter so prettily on my sleeve was guarded more preciously than any earthly treasure. Hurt, pain or sadness, each had a place to hide where light of day could not penetrate and expose the wound. In a sense then I would be invulnerable, always the strong one, balanced and wise. It fooled us both – for a while…

The trouble was, invulnerable people don't get cancer.

The statue was crumbling, tumbling bit-by-bit from its ivory pedestal and exposing beneath its polished, perfect stone the soft pink frailty of humanity. I had, of course, always known what lay within, had had my family to cry with when the pain was too hot to hold safely inside, the sadness too big to squeeze into its tiny cupboard. Still, I never told Ben; instead I left it to the enemy, to the cancer to rise up, lisping slyly at his ear, and tell him that I was vulnerable after all and that it was only a matter of time…

He wasn't, they said, to come close, to kiss or hold me, for risk of passing on infection – the steely-eyed sister kept stern vigil as she passed outside the two small windows that looked out onto the ward outside my room. So he closed the blinds and lay still and quiet beside me, resolutely defying the policing as if in doing so he was defying the very disease that stole through my veins. And she opened them again and thrust reality, along with the harsh fluorescent light, back into our little room, reminding us that the threat was real and that even a cold could take my fading life and not return it.

When, after the fourth week they let me home for a time, a concession in the guise of a reprieve whereby I had to journey each day to the hospital for my chemotherapy, he was always there.

In the mornings he would lift me into the car, as if across the threshold, and for a while we were bound for the sea, the forest or a glitzy theme park of candy-floss, roller coasters and frivolity. And then we arrived and there were needles and pain and poisons, and when our salty sea breeze swept through my hair it carried the soft fair strands with it, choking and blinding us both as it went.

In the evenings, when we hid in my room, the demons came out to dance. Shrieking and mocking they danced, trampling on all that was familiar and real. With their hard, pointed feet and long spiny talons they rent and tore at the little floral curtains that brushed the deep-set window-seat, they split open the soft lumpy cushions of the friendly old sofa that hugged the ancient chimney-breast opposite my bed. They swung, in their frenzy, from the low uneven beams; cast new, unfamiliar shadows across the room whose face had always been as much a part of me as my own. And we could only watch, Ben and I, as we lay there, he atop the covers, me beneath. To the casual eye my big attic bedroom might appear just as it had always done, warm, cosy and cheerful with just the right scattering of untidy, but we knew better. We knew that nothing was truly just as it had always been... or would ever be so again.

They got inside our minds too, the demons, warping and distorting our fragile inner world. We could hear them laughing as they added yet more bricks to the wall which loomed up so indomitable between us and mocked our ever more hopeless struggles to surmount its height and touch the other side. Their biggest joke was the denial that seemed to grip Ben with sudden, indiscriminate zeal. The rough, forbidden kisses that he stole paid no heed to hidden dangers, to the legions of deadly bacteria that lurked in the wings; his veiled eyes were blinded to the vast swathes of baby blond that came away in his hands with each passionate caress. My heart reached out and the terror pulled me back. In vain I sought to find him, to seek that place to which he ran, where nothing was expected of us but to be young, reckless and in love, but my pain-wracked body tied me too fast to the realm of the demons.

And thus we flailed, lost and alone. And never was the

isolation more painful than in our last desperate attempts to bring down that wall before we lost sight of each other forever…

We did try.

But it was stronger than we were…

Chapter Twenty Three
The Secret

If I tell you about the night They almost beat me will you promise to keep my secret? If you give them an inch, so the saying goes, and the Demons have already stolen too much of my life. Still they must have known they had the upper hand. After all, the doctors had been so clear and earnest about what it meant too for me to be neutropaenic. My immune system, they told me, was completely destroyed. Consequently I had no resistance to infection, even a common cold could kill me.

All around me in the shadows the Demons' ears pricked up.

Strangely, though, this was all part of the plan. A kind of training programme to shock the wayward cells back into line. A 'kill or cure' tactic. We just had to hope the Demons didn't call our bluff. Infection, the doctors continued, was inevitable. The critical thing was to catch it coming, before it had a chance to take a hold. Like, I thought, discerning the cloud before the rain, the wind before the storm. Ensuring you are curled up safely by the fireside when the drops begin to fall.

Only here it wasn't just about getting wet. From the moment my temperature began to rise in response to an invader every second counted. If I was not treated with intravenous antibiotics within twenty minutes of the clouds gathering... The Demon cackle rose to a roar and the foot of the curtain swayed in anticipation of that first gust of wind.

So, there I was, utterly vulnerable to even the most benign of the bug world, and stuck in a hospital, surrounded by every disease known to man and quite possibly a good many more they were yet to become acquainted with. Ironic, eh? And whilst those fetching polythene accessories had been good for a laugh, I was not, when my life was on the line, altogether persuaded as to their having earnt such a frontline position in my army. I had wanted to go home.

If infection was inevitable then I would rather catch a cold from my brother than Polynesian Bird Flu from, well, er, a Polynesian bird. The only snag was that home was, on an optimistic day, a good twenty minutes from the hospital. Mummy was under strict instruction. My temperature would have to be taken every fifteen minutes, night and day, to monitor the slightest change. At the earliest sign, night or day, I would have to be rushed in to hospital post haste or be dead as a doornail within minutes. Not your most popular houseguest. Still, my family loved me and my room had never looked so wonderful as it did that day when Daddy carried me home.

But then the clouds came. We didn't need the thermometer to tell us they were coming. The fever built with terrifying rapidity.

The 'life or death' journey to the hospital passed me by in an anguished haze of pain and confusion. Bourne on Angels' wings my astonishing mother flew through the night, the dark clouds looming and the wind whipping at our heels. Until we were there. But instead of the hypnotic warmth of the fireside and a large mug of cocoa there were harsh strip lights, shadows to hide the Demons – and those needles. Needles to force into tiny veins that screamed with each aborted attempt. Needles that warped and stretched in my fevered imagination. Needles that, though every atom of my being cried out against them, were all that stood between me and the end of my war.

And all around me lay the wounded and the dying. My isolation room was unavailable with our having arrived without warning and my bed was just one among many, distinguished merely by it's position in the pool of cold blue light that illuminated the nurse's station. My nameless, faceless companions in the field were discernable only by the moans that came periodically out of the shadows, lonely and devoid of hope. I clung as though my life depended on it – and it did – to Mummy's hand. In her was my link to the other world. Confirmation that it was there that I truly belonged. The gateway back to the land of the living.

And then they took her away. And it wasn't the Demons but the hard, brusque Agency Nurse who took away my lifeline, insisted that Mummy must surely need to rest, and could come back tomorrow. And the anguish on Mummy's face equalled mine as they tore us apart and the Demons escorted her triumphantly out of the ward.

We knew that tomorrow might be too late.

And, as I lay there alone in the gloaming, almost blind with a raging fever and the pain that seared through my very soul, the most terrifying thing of all was that I couldn't care anymore. If the battle was over then I was ready to surrender. I just wanted to close my eyes and for it all to be over. But God wasn't ready for me that night. Instead He took the old man from the bed beside mine. So, He, like me, had heard the pleas for help that sounded pitifully through the night. He, unlike the nurses, had answered the call.

And as I sat up and greeted the new day, the pain and fever vanquished and Mummy's quick steps sounding in the corridor, I knew that, just for a moment, as He passed, He had paused by the bed next door.

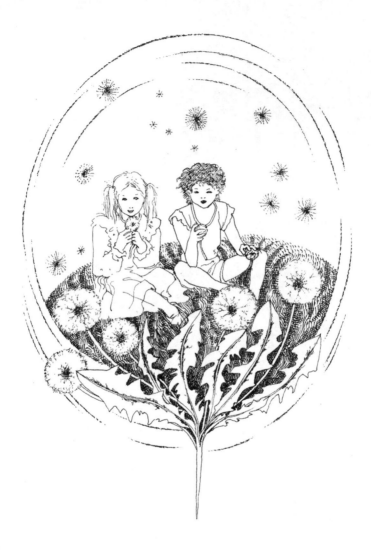

"Dandelions are what rabbits like best."

114

Chapter Twenty Four

Amy

They do say that it is in times of trouble that you find out who your real friends are. Well, if there was ever a time of trouble then I guess this was it. And if there was ever a real friend then it must be Amy.

What 'me and Amy' liked doing best was feeding the rabbits. We always asked old Mrs Ragg, (she was, we guessed, more than 100 years old), before we picked the dandelions that flourished so magnificently along her verdant driveway. Dandelions are what rabbits like best. And, since we always asked so very politely…

And sometimes what we liked doing best was playing games; and sometimes it was counting the small shiny beetles that ambled precariously over the lush, bendy blades of grass, or numbering the big black spots on the tomato-red back of the friendly ladybird. And sometimes it was 'piggy-back' races on all fours in the garden with her sister Claire and with Jeremy. And sometimes it was picnics in the forest and sometimes it was going to the zoo…

And sometimes what we liked best of all was being three and three-quarters instead of only three.

When she visited me that day in the hospital - during those first two weeks when the world was still spinning and I hid, for safety, behind my big brick wall - she brought with her a vast photo album, plump and shiny with our earliest memories. She spread it open across my lap and we pointed and chuckled and remembered.

At least that is what she told me later. I wasn't there at the time. But I am so glad that she was.

Amy was there the very first time I went to the hospital. That time I was the patient too and Amy was the nurse who administered the large wooden bead into my right nostril, all ready for Dr Claire to operate on and remove. Unfortunately it happened that Dr Claire was equipped with neither the implements nor the skills to perform such delicate surgery and thus we were obliged to call upon a very nice man in A&E and I had to promise Mummy I would never do anything so silly again.

Not long after that Big Adventure, I was going to have another one, but this time without Claire and Amy. In fact, after the day we packed up all our things and moved away from that little house with mustard and cress on the windowsill and my two best friends just around the corner, I didn't see them very often at all. Still, our mothers kept in touch and every now and then, at Easter or at half term, I would go and visit, and eat chocolate eggs and go on bicycle rides and have adventures... until some time when I was about twelve, and after that there were really only rememberings...

But when rememberings are as good as ours were you can never really forget. Though our subsequent lives had carried us along such different streams, if you followed the rushing water back down-stream for far enough you would always come back to an overgrown driveway and four little hands clutching dandelion leaves as if they were manna from heaven...

Amy's first letter arrived two days after her visit. The bright red envelope marked it out most theatrically from the others in the pile and I drew the enclosed sheet from within with heightened curiosity. Written on the equally startling page in a slightly awkward hand was a poem and, nestled in between the naively gentle lines, was Amy's heart.

I knew little about the troubles that Amy had gone through in the six or seven years since we had seen each other, but I knew enough to know that this open, simple expression of love was the greatest gift that anyone could ever give. As the tears that had, until then, remained so tightly locked away flowed freely down my cheeks I gave my heart right back to Amy and knew that, for the first time since I built my wall, I had a friend who was truly on my side...

The second letter arrived the very next day; and the third the day after that. And, as the weeks became months, it was with eager, happy fingers that I tore into the bright red envelope that arrived each morning, long after the first flood of other cards had become a merest trickle.

And at other times, in the darkest hours when the demons were dancing and Terror incited me to hide away from the rest of the world, there was Amy, who through two hundred sheets of bright red paper showed me all I know about what it is to be a friend...

Chapter Twenty Five

Jim

You know how it is in a dream when you reach the end of a winding corridor, fling open the door in front of you and are not remotely taken aback to find a tap-dancing pig playing the bugle or your third-year history master in galoshes knitting a twenty-three foot scarf out of cold spaghetti?

Well, the lines between waking and sleep had become well and truly blurred as far as I was concerned and consequently my realm of experience broke down neatly into three categories, namely; 'bizarre/bad'; 'bizarre/good' and just plain 'bizarre'…Anything vaguely 'normal' might have knocked me down with a feather but otherwise I was totally unshockable.

Thus, one fine, surreal morn, (three weeks or so into my sentence), as I lay, drugged up to the eyeballs, in my minimalist boudoir, I batted not an eyelid at the unannounced arrival of Sir James Saville OBE – plus copious amounts of gold jewellery and very distinctly minus the fetching polythene accoutrements that were essential garb for mere mortal visitors. (I guessed that famous people didn't harbour bacteria). Given that, in fact, for the next twelve hours or so, my eyelids were about the only part of my anatomy that I was permitted to move, as I had just undergone a particularly grim procedure after which any significant movement might induce irreparable brain damage, (hey…ho), I doubtless appeared somewhat under-whelmed to see him. Still, since he generated more than enough pomp and ceremony for the both of us it is doubtful that he noticed.

As to which of the three current realms of experience this arrival fell into, I was not altogether sure at the outset. With a 'jangle, jangle' of 'jewellery, jewellery' and with a hefty whiff of cigar smoke following in his wake, in bounced one of the foremost of my childhood heroes, swiftly and simperingly followed by an entourage of nursing staff all eager to cop sight of my reaction. Quite what they were anticipating given the heavily enforced restrictions on my movement I am not entirely sure but, failing the colourful Irish jig, I put on my broadest smile and hoped that I didn't disappoint.

In truth, anything that provided a distraction from the whole 'brain damage' bit was a welcome diversion and, since ordinarily my daily 'news', when it came down to entertaining my parents of an evening, tended to rely rather too heavily on how many mls. of urine I had managed to pass or whether my haemoglobin count was up or down, there was no doubt that I could do with some new material. And so, I concluded, this narrowed it down to 'bizarre/ good' or just plain 'bizarre'; as to which was more apt, I had no doubt I was about to find out...

To be frank, naked and horizontal, (although at least still at that stage in possession of my hair), would not have been my preferred choice for meeting anyone, but, since making a dash for it seemed very much off the cards, I inched the covers up a little higher and resolved to make the best of things.

I had long been aware that when Sir Jim was not making small people's dreams come true one was very likely to find him at Stoke Mandeville. Here, at the world renowned National Spinal Injuries Centre, the wish list that had confronted him for more than thirty years was in striking contrast to the prime-time one of pop bands, helicopter rides and sweet factories. Where the anguished prayer of a young traffic-accident victim was for feeling in his shattered, limp and useless limbs, to be able to walk, run and play football once more, or simply to be able to bath, dress and feed himself, Jim knew better than anyone that there were no strings to pull, no instant 'fixes'. Instead there were years of intense emotional and physical therapy, there was anger and pain, hopelessness and despair, and, thanks to tireless fund-raising and publicity by Jim and his team, there was the Stoke Mandeville Spinal Injuries Centre and there was hope…

In gracing the less hallowed halls of ward 1X, however, the cabbage (as it were) was very much away from its patch, and I have to confess to just a twinge of 'chuffed-ness' in learning from a beaming Sister Watson that this visit was exclusively on my account. Not at all sure that I could, in my present state, live up to the enormous honour that was clearly being bestowed, I nevertheless smiled gamely and suppressed the urge to berate my caller for all those letters that he never answered. Still, I conceded, a personal visit kind of made up for his past rudeness.

And it wasn't to be just the one. From that day onwards, it seemed, Sir James never left. The strange, if not to say 'bizarre', thing was we hit it off. Behind the closed door of my little room the flamboyant showman laid down his top hat and we talked; really talked. For the first time since the sky had fallen in, there was someone curious to know what it was like for a young, active girl to be living with cancer, as opposed to dying from it. I could talk about my future, about the hopes and dreams that I would make reality when the Nightmare released me from its underworld domain. And I could laugh and joke and know that the twinge of pain that might, now and then, show on my face would not ricochet through my companion like a bullet…

And if those hours spent with Mr Fix-It in hospital were surreal, then those spent outside it were to be positively fantastical. But that's another story...stay tuned!

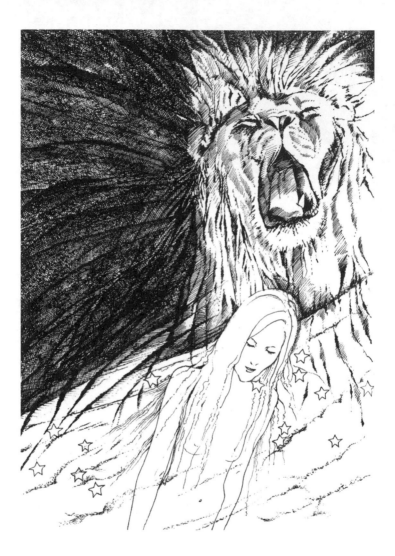

"Only by facing the Demons might I exile them once and for all."

Chapter Twenty Six

Hades

The danger, people say, of long-term hospitalisation, is that one becomes 'institutionalised', afraid to leave the safety of its eternally whitewashed walls for the multi-coloured world without. As I lay there each day, my soul crying out for the thirst-quenching green of the natural world, the blue/grey of the sky, the rose-pink scent of the honeysuckle below my bedroom window and the warm, golden caress of the late autumn sun, such a concept was incomprehensible. The Demons could build their wall a thousand feet high and I would always scale it, fight my way back to the world beyond, the world in which I truly belonged. Of that I was certain.

How could I have known that in those few weeks since Pluto first carried me down, down, down into the dark, the world I knew before had been changing. Over its once friendly visage, so safe, comforting and familiar, an evil spell had been wrought, rendering it terrifyingly unpredictable and harsh, so loud and chaotic as to leave me reeling. It was not even a month since I had left - but the Demons work quickly…

I had been so excited about our shopping trip. Mummy was concerned that it might be too much for me, but she could see the sparkle in my eyes and had to acknowledge that I was in need of something to wear during my brief sojourn home that didn't hang off my frail new form like the borrowed coat of a scarecrow. So it was with a happy heart, albeit too with the somewhat wobbly, unpredictable gait of a new-born colt, that I pushed open the doors of the little Benetton store and reassured Mummy that I would be fine for a few minutes whilst she popped in to the shop next door. Five minutes later I emerged, triumphant and resplendent in Benetton's finest jeans and jumper combination and with Mummy nowhere to be seen.

And then I had a good idea and the world fell in.

It wasn't until I was deeply submerged among the shelves and aisles of the vast Boots store that was, after all, only a stone's throw across the way, that the Demons played their trump card. Having conjured so cunningly the illusion that both the world and I were as of old, that our relationship was one of mutual respect and understanding, it was with cackles of glee that they tore away the veil. As the noise and chaos built around me, so the aisles began to sway and buckle. The mountains of jars, bottles, packets and bags merged into a nauseating blur of colour and form, looming and swirling under the harsh glare of the overhead light. The people around me, their own pre-set course warped by the evil spell, began to fight and jostle, jolting and knocking against my screaming bones as I stood paralysed and waited for the end of the world to play out its final chord…

And then, somehow, I was staggering and reeling towards the doors, any knowledge of what had originally lured me so unwittingly into the demons' lair utterly vanquished from my mind in the all-consuming urge for survival. And there was Mummy, sweeping me into her arms with a relieved sigh, and the Demons departed, screeching and wailing their frustrations as they went.

But I knew they were out there just waiting for a chance to catch me alone…

In truth I didn't feel safe anywhere. Contrary to the

psychiatrist's musings, the fact that the outside world seemed alien and unpredictable did not automatically render the hospital world of routine and predictability safe and appealing. However challenging my experiences beyond the walls, it was my experiences within that strained at the very boundaries of courage and fear.

Thus that final night at home, before the devil called in his deal and I returned to the second bout of 'intensification' therapy, was tortuous beyond describing. In general, I would always argue that it is the 'unknown' that is the most terrifying enemy of all. Where chemotherapy is concerned, the knowing takes one beyond all imaginings. This time, as I prepared to step into the arena, to confront the lions unarmed and naked, I knew the strength of their roar, the power of their claws, the sharpness of their teeth…and I was afraid. The enemy was not my leukaemia, the struggling, sick cells that I knew fought so bravely to right themselves and heal, but the hospital machine that, cold and impersonal, threatened to taunt and beat me until I broke and it spat me out, another casualty of its pointless, gratuitous war against humanity and the soul. To give myself up to that enemy without a fight went against all my deepest instincts.

As I pleaded with Jeremy not to let them take me back, I knew that he would not let me down. We had a pact, an unspoken deal born out of seventeen years of bickering and rivalries, mischief and love, that said that we would always be there for each other. If the outside world took on one of us then it was taking on us both. This was one battle that neither of us, vulnerable and afraid, knew how to fight, but there was no doubt that when the bell sounded we would be standing in the same corner - fists up. Huddled together that night, in the warm pocket of light cast by my little bedside lamp, tears steaming down our faces and hands tightly clasped, we may not have appeared all that invincible, but when you have love on your side then your strength knows no bounds…

But this time, even as he made his promise, both he and I knew deep down that the only chance we had of truly winning lay in my offering myself up at the lion's mouth. It was the first of December, five weeks after I slipped into borrowed time. It was the beginning of Advent and with God on my side I left home for the battle of my life.

Only by facing the demons might I exile them once and for all.

Chapter Twenty Seven
The Wooden Horse

Their armoury was a fearsome one. Already they had fortune on their side. An unfortunate accident when administering a shot of chemotherapy had seen the toxic chemicals leak insidiously out of my punctured vein and flood mercilessly into the vulnerable tissue of my right arm. The huge, swollen limb that hung uselessly and agonisingly from my shoulder was unrecognisable as my own. The vast weeping blister that formed as the tissue continued to burn from the inside out was further testimony to the heinous nature of the drugs that were assailing my body from all sides. And these poisonous, creeping chemicals were supposed to be on my team? They were the frontline in my army? As the doctors discussed my potential need for plastic surgery on the damaged arm, I retreated further behind my wall, reassured in the knowledge that it was now so high that even the Demons would have a hard time finding me.

But I had underestimated their cunning. Just as the Greeks sent their wooden horse into Troy, so the Demons hid expectantly in the wings as their own secret weapon invaded my room. I lay there, cradling my grotesquely bulbous arm in a rolled blanket, awaiting the arrival of my next shot of chemo, when the nurse came in, wheeling before her a skeletal form, death staring out from its darkly sunken eyes. Male or female? One couldn't tell. Behind her staggered the foot soldiers, pained and weary in their ongoing battle to remain this side of death. Eyes wide in horror and grief at such evident hopeless suffering, I clenched my fingers hard into my palm to remind myself to hold on, to keep from releasing the long, anguished scream which resonated through every fibre of my inner being. Then came the poisoned arrow.

"You see how lucky you are?" the nurse enquired breezily of the living dead. "You could be Emma."

The odd thing is that, despite a good deal of overwhelming evidence to the contrary, I never felt like I 'had leukaemia'. The endless days and nights alone and traumatised in my hospital room were instead a kind of nonsensical mistake; the young people around me who were 'terminally sick' were to be sympathised with and admired for their courage but I was not 'one of them'. Perhaps it was a form of disassociation, orchestrated by my mind to protect itself from confronting the possibility of dying. Perhaps it was, as I felt at times, God within me, reassuring me that it was not my time to go, but I certainly never considered myself to be the proverbial 'victim' of a terminal disease. I was just me. Perhaps in my ignorance I had been guilty of 'categorising' the sick, elderly or disabled into homogenous groups, defining them not as individuals but instead imposing my own narrow-minded presumptions upon them. Perhaps we are all just 'us', doing the best we can to stay afloat with whatever life throws our way? Perhaps too there are those who find a kind of security or companionship in 'belonging' to such a 'group', who find that their illness gives them a kind of 'identity', even 'importance', that their lives have previously lacked? Who am I to say? It is hard enough to fathom one's own complex and extraordinary responses to a world that has suddenly turned tail overnight and reneged on all that it had promised. But I do know that somewhere beneath all the drips and tubes I was still just me.

Had I been able to comprehend, deep down, the life-depending necessity of the oh-so-brutal treatment regime, perhaps the horror would have been easier to bear.

Or perhaps not.

Sometimes I think that the endless nights were the worst, but then I remember the days and I am not so sure. Day or night, marking out the slow steady crawl of each agonising minute as it passed, was the clock that loomed mockingly down from the wall opposite my bed. What a strange idea to hang a clock, the only feature in a stark, bare room, directly in the patient's eye-line. Might one wish to count down one's final hours; reflect, as each hour sounds its passing, upon all the time that will never come again; time that has been irretrievably lost in the deprivation of a real world in which it actually has some meaning other than the steady tick, tick of a cold grey dial?

Ironically, still more tortuous was my gradual, creeping inability to read that dial. As, day-by-day, the once all too crisp, clear numbers blurred to a series of increasingly indistinct smudges, the clock became a terrifying yardstick by which to measure the dramatic decline of my sight. In this world where horror knew no bounds, I knew that it was only a matter of time before I was completely blind, trapped forever in the darkness which breathed ever more heavily at my heels...

To know it was one thing; to hear it said was another. So I stayed quiet when the doctors came into my room, held my fears wrapped tightly around my chest where they crushed and choked me with their slow, insidious squeeze. Instead of fearing death I feared the eternal dark. Each time the door-handle turned I was sure that it heralded the imminent arrival of a casual comment, tossed out as a 'by-the-way'; a "by-the-way, we forgot to mention that you are going blind", sort of comment to hang alongside the "by-the-way, you will lose all your hair", memo; the "by-the-way, you are unlikely to be able to have children", post-script, and the ('if they didn't get to you, maybe this will'), "by-the-way, these drugs might kill you", foot-note. I dreaded, continually, the visit of a porter with his empty wheelchair, all set to run me this time, not to the X-Ray department to monitor the development of my cancer, but to the eye specialist to monitor the development of my blindness. I was terrified by my fears but still more terrified to have them confirmed, so I just waited, squinted and waited, and prayed that God knew that there was only so much that I could take…

I talked to Him mostly in the night-time. Night-time in the underworld isn't black with tiny silver pin-pricks of stars. Night-time here is a shivery grey, a cold, sad gloaming, presided over by a single fluorescent bulb that allows one neither the ability to fully wake or sleep. And so I talked to God; and to myself. And because I found God there inside me, it was the same thing. And as I stroked the soft, warm skin on my long, thin arm, in between the drip tubes and needles, it was so alive. And God told me not to be afraid; He reminded me of all the trillions of cells, all the ones that I could see and all those that I couldn't, that resounded with that life, and that were not going to relinquish their hold on it without a fight.

I could feel them fighting. Sometimes when I thought hard enough I could feel each individual cell, quivering with the life that was going to triumph over death. Alone in that little room I could hear my thoughts shouting through the thin grey light. My breathing was so large and important that I could have been breathing for a whole battalion, not just for me. And then my breathing was so large and important that I forgot how to do it and lay there in the shadows wondering if instead that was what would finally get me, simply forgetting how to live...

But there was always someone there to remind me. Every fifteen minutes, night and day, someone was there to take my 'obs.', or 'observations', my pulse, temperature and blood pressure, just to make sure that I hadn't forgotten. And so I didn't sleep but I did keep breathing.

If they were happy that I was still alive then they would give me a little more of what might kill me, just to push our luck. Silhouetted against the door in the strange unearthly light, the night-doctor, armed with his poisonous syringe was all your childhood demons made one. Each night he had a different face, looming over mine in the gloom, as, with a cold, perfunctory detachment, he performed his task and left, taking with him another part of my soul and leaving behind the damp and clinging shroud of fear...

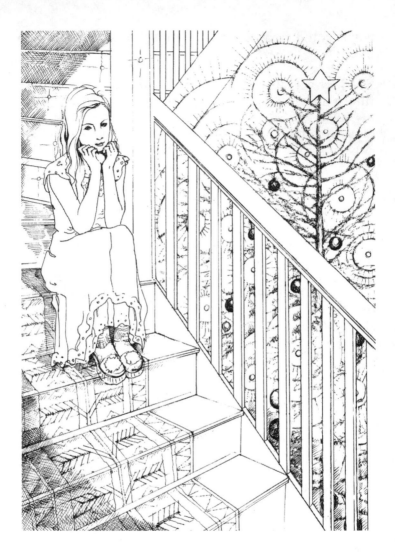

"...I could feel the air shimmering with the power of The Christmas Miracle."

Chapter Twenty Eight
Advent

Anyway, for better or worse, there I was, three weeks before Christmas and wondering if it would be my last.

I had certainly had more than my fair share of magical Christmases. Naturally since God lived in our house, the birth of His only begotten Son was always an occasion for a jolly good 'knees up'. Our rambling Georgian home did the Victorian family Christmas thing magnificently, and the fact that there were so many of us to sing angelically around the huge, bedecked tree added still further to the all-round authenticity. Admittedly the vast swathes of enthusiastically draped, multi-coloured tinsel and the increasingly neurotic string of plastic fairy lights, (now-you see-them-now-you-don't), owed more to Mr Woolworth than Charles Dickens, but candles had been rejected early on – it seems that when it comes to fire hazards, dodgy wiring is as far as Daddy is prepared to go. So we would feast and sing and pray and nervously practise readings for the carol service and, when we had half a chance, slip furtively into the 'television room' with pockets full of Quality Street to watch re-runs of Morecambe and Wise (or, indeed, whatever happened to be on) and be secretly glad that there were some things that we did even better than the Victorians.

So far this year I felt somewhat let down. My advent calendar was there, propped up beside my bed and there was Mummy beside me frantically writing Christmas cards; but it wasn't my bed and with each word she wrote I could feel Mummy shrink a little inside as she passed on our 'Christmas news'.

Just outside my window a 'Christmas raffle' table had been set up which, whilst not exactly lending an air of festive 'bonhomie', at least gave Mummy and me a giggle as we observed the steady trickle of gloomy faces peer beyond the ubiquitous bottle of whisky into my room and speculated whether I might be considered the first or second prize… Mummy and I had become rather good at our own form of black humour. It's amazing what makes you laugh if it means one less thing to cry about.

Still, though the odds admittedly did not appear stacked in its favour, I was determined that the spirit of Christmas should win through. Christmas, I had known since a little girl, was about much more than just exciting shaped parcels, flame-haloed plum puddings and tangerine filled stocking toes; it was about Miracles. At nights, I would sit at the top of our broad, winding staircase and look down on the wondrous tree that lit the vast hallway below with its soft, rainbow light and I could feel the air shimmering with the power of The Christmas Miracle. Even wars, someone had told me at a very impressionable age, were halted in its mysterious wake, and if it could stop, even for a moment, the senseless brutality of war then its power was without limits. In the face of such an immutable force, fear and pain were surely inconsequential; the combined miracles of love and joy, miracles that my short life had been blessed with in abundance, could rise and conquer all.

And knowing that I had The Miracle on my side made me stronger. And, in between the needles and the vomiting, Mummy, my brave, extraordinary mother, and I made plans for a truly wonderful Christmas. In the dark hours I would picture, excitedly, the intrigued, happy faces of those I loved beyond comprehension, as they tore away the cheerful wrappings that hid the little well-thought out surprises that I was arranging from my hospital bed. I looked forward impatiently to the week when all the family - aunts, uncles, cousins and grandparents – would come together once again and celebrate the privilege of love and joy and miracles...

(And eat too much).

And in the meantime Daddy and I would fill this sad little room with carols and giggling and funny stories, and Mummy and I would laugh and cry and find ways to free our spirits from the confines of the walls and of unspoken dread... Once we really broke out, slipped our moorings and, before the ward sister could come upon us, dashed mischievously to the car, my rose-pink satin slippers click-clicking conspiratorially on the tarmac. Then, as we sat, minutes later, in the sweeping gravel drive of a nearby pub, a ploughman's lunch had never tasted so delicious and Mummy's sherry was liquid gold because for that moment we were free and life was still out there, waiting...

The world of the (potentially!) terminally ill is an exclusive one. Never in my most tortured dreams could I have conjured such a place of suffering and pain. Had I done so though, I know without a doubt that I could not have imagined the glory of its redemption. There was a window here in this place of darkness and despair and through it shone a courage, beauty and inner peace that left the Demons blinded and reeling in its light and left me humbled and in awe. Skimming blithely across the surface of the old world how unaware I had been of its hidden secrets. How ironic it is that with so much to teach us, the sick and injured and dying are rushed and huddled into their underworld domain, as far from those of us who have so much to learn as is possible.

For me this astonishing, guiding 'light' will always have a name: Simon. Sometimes when I looked out of my large, internal window onto the corridor beyond, I caught sight of an old man shuffling painfully along, head bowed and back stooped with the weight of his years. He was, I had guessed by his parched, wrinkled skin and thin, white wispy hair and flaking scalp, well over eighty years old. His name, Mummy said, was Simon and he often asked about me. He was gentle and kind and made her smile. He sent books too, though for risk of cross-infection Mummy was obliged to keep them safely in her handbag for a while and then return them with our warmest wishes. Simon had a rare form of leukaemia and he 'lived' in the other isolation room, next to mine; he had been there for seven years. Mummy had sat and talked with him often and, yes, with his mother.

Simon, you see, was only nineteen years old. Still now I think of Simon often – though I never even had the chance to say 'hello'. When the road feels particularly long and rocky, Simon is there, smiling reassuringly and reminding me that, though my limbs may become weary, at each step, with courage and faith, my spirit need grow only stronger…

Chapter Twenty Nine
One More Corner

Early on I realised that the only way to tackle that road really was step by step. To attempt the journey with a continual awareness of the many miles that still lay ahead, the hazards and the pitfalls that threatened to steer me off my course, might leave me floundering, exhausted and afraid, at the roadside before I had even begun.

My treatment regime was divided conveniently into its various courses; 'induction', 'intensification', 'maintenance', etc; and, rather than look beyond the current reign of terror to the unimaginable horrors of the next, I resolved to conquer each new mountain as if it were not merely one of a huge and insurmountable range. The end would always be just around the corner.

Daddy had taught us this most valuable philosophy at a very early point in our childhood – indeed on a particularly memorable occasion involving a long car journey, two grumpy children and copious amounts of sick (Jeremy's, I hasten to make clear, rather than mine). Suffice to say we all learnt that day not only the power of positive thinking but also the wisdom that sometimes in life 'the s***' well and truly 'hits the fan' anyway and, philosophy or no, you just have to get down on your hands and knees and clear it up.

Anyway, as things now stood, some twelve years on, I was hoping to draw upon this dual wisdom to see me through – and so far I certainly had the requisite amount of vomit!

For now then I resolved to see my way until my Christmas 'break'. Looming dark and threatening on the post-Christmas horizon was the terrifying spectre of Radiotherapy and to anticipate that alongside managing the 'intensification' block was inconceivable if I were to keep the demons from running riot.

How strange it was to recall for a moment a parallel universe in which I might be setting off for my Oxford interviews this very week, my head full of 'dreaming spires', Thomas Hardy and punting on the Cherwell. Like that of the archetypal Dickensian street urchin, peering in through the half-open shutters of the 'big' house as inside its inhabitants laughed and danced, feasted and made merry, my heart yearned for the golden-hued world that lay just the other side of the wall - even as my head told me that it was a world of which I could forever only dream…Once upon a time there was a girl who flew to America; who spread her wings and soared on the new wind; who read Bronte and munched carrot cake on the harbour wall; who danced on the beach with the incoming tide and who knew that this was only the beginning…How strange that I could almost touch her, could almost feel her heart beat, think her thoughts, dream her dreams and yet she was forever just beyond my reach.

And then I knew that whatever it took I would find her and I would find the light in all the darkness to guide my way. I would dance her dance once more and my feet would never after touch the ground because I knew now that the music in this world doesn't go on forever and you have to hear and harness it like sails in the wind and know that it is a gift to use finely and with all your heart and soul…

And then it was Christmas and I was going home.

Chapter Thirty

Christmas

The floor of my brightly lit bedroom was a garden, resplendent – one might even say riotous – with colour; bejewelled, bedecked, bestrewn. In amidst the glory sat my Aunt Jane, Hannah and my small cousin Kate, a large pair of scissors and the Spirit of Christmas. Crackers were well and truly 'in progress' and though this year I could only watch as the reams of coloured paper, tinsel and balloons came together in an unashamedly kitsch harmony of ruffles and bows, the sense of tradition and ceremony was no less diminished. I was home and cradled in the arms of familiarity and enterprise; the bright shouts of laughter at a potential 'motto' and the occasional urgent requests to "pass the scissors" filled the room with hope in the way that only 'normality' can and my thirsty soul drank in all that it could in preparation for the long, dry journey that awaited just over the brow…

Whilst my soul drank in the normality, my body, it seemed, couldn't get enough of minced beef. Which was just as well since, when incited into combat with the Aga, my intrepid grandmother who, for better or worse had gamely stepped into the breach for a while, was reduced to a one-dish menu; Shepherd's Pie. Such was my capacity for this rustic fare that the table each evening was laden down with not one but two large pies, one for everyone else and one for me. My body too was making the most of this oasis and if cravings are anything to go by it seemed to know exactly what it needed. Except for one slightly dubious occasion, (which I put down not a little nervously to a combination of enforced hospital fare and a surfeit of similarly enforced hallucinogenic drugs), on which my father's fingers took on the decidedly irresistible guise of a plate of sausages, I felt I could pretty much trust its instincts. Subsequently each day I tucked, with astonishing zeal, into a great proportion of the world's food mountains of beef-steak, broccoli-cheese and Brussels sprouts. Doubtless a nutritionist would mumble meaningful insights about iron content and the like but all I knew was that they tasted DELICIOUS. The novelty too of consuming a meal without having to bring it all up again a short while later had not escaped my notice and this I meant to do justice to in the finest of manners.

So there I was, feasting and laughing, and things were altogether looking up. To cap it all I had my hair back. At least, I had someone else's hair back, but believe me beggars can't be choosers and when whoever's I had was as bountiful and glamorous as this then who cared?

My new flowing locks were altogether thanks to Heather. Her visit to one of London's premier wig-makers, armed with a skein of my 'old' hair for colour match, had yielded nothing short of a miracle. This was not hair for shrinking violets. This hair undulated and flowed, glistened and gleamed - all the way down to my bottom! And, as I discovered on subsequent nerve-wracking forays into the 'real' world, it cried out to be caressed. What was more, compared with the more traditional, one might even say commonplace, kind that grows out of your head, this hair was decidedly low maintenance, no small bonus when for 90% of the time one is accompanied at insensitively close quarters by large, unwieldy metal drip stands – Joan Collins and Dolly Parton were clearly wiser than I might have in the past surmised. It's true that when sporting said 'cascade' I bore more than a passing resemblance to a well-known brand of doll, but since this seemed to enamour me greatly to my hitherto extremely shy five-year-old cousin Kate I figured this was no bad thing.

Trying out my new look on the outside world was another matter entirely. It was with a heart-pumping blend of excitement and blind terror that I climbed out of the car outside the cinema with my friend Sally – and it was not entirely accountable for by her having mistaken a quiet country drive for some kind of extreme sport – (and one, let me tell you, nerve-wrackingly akin to hang-gliding).

The Point multi-screen cinema with its bars and restaurants loomed large and brash – entertainment Vegas-style and we loved it. My black felt trilby sat jauntily atop my new crowning glory and I reached up momentarily to feel the reassurance of its presence before, with a squeeze of Sally's hand, I stepped through the doors. After months in a small grey room with little sound other than the ticking of the clock it was like Armageddon. An ambush of music and light assailed me from all sides, pulsing through the very core of my being, absorbing me into its living, breathing, amorphic form even as my eyes were still adjusting to its ever-changing face. It was terrifying and WONDERFUL and I was ALIVE!

And then I was sashaying down the central aisle, holding my head up high to hide the fact that I was really bald and naked. And when the boys asked to buy me a drink I accepted an orange-juice graciously and when they asked flirtatiously if they could try on my hat and smiled even as they stretched out to strip me of my black felt courage, I smiled back coyly - and moved just a little further out of reach.

And when we drove home again we laughed, Sally and I; how we laughed. And suddenly my wall was only three feet high instead of twelve and, if I screwed up my eyes tight and made a giant leap, I might even have stepped over it into the old world – just for a while...

What can I tell you about Sally except that she was a part of me? She was beautiful and brilliant, anxious and honest – and she took hours in the bathroom before we went out. She showed me that the old world was still there and guided me across the threshold; she laughed with me and cried with me and took the world upon her shoulders. But even as she coaxed me back into that big, bright, colourful world she was recoiling from it herself; into a deep, dark, terrible place where only I could find her.

And she knew that we needed salvation. So she got on a plane and went to Israel to try and save the world. But instead she picked water melons with an army of other disillusioned heroes. Until her soul was bleached out with her hair and the earth was just a round green ball full of pips and with no hope for the future. And God saw that that was no way for her to live.

That morning was different. That morning the telephone didn't ring.

You could hear it from my room when it rang – along the corridor, (and a little wiggle). And you could hear when it didn't. I listened hard for it's shrill, echoey call as if that might make it all the more likely to come. But it didn't. Six a.m., then seven, eight, nine did come and go – and Reason's voice wasn't loud enough to fill the quiet that swelled my head and squeezed my heart. Until he got impatient with not being heard and told me to go and make that call. And then I was there in that little alcove under the windy stone staircase, the money tinkling down into the box, the big black receiver cold and greasy in my hand. "Is Sally there?," I asked politely of the silence that picked up the receiving end. More silence. So much silence that morning. Then, just when I thought that there was no sound worse than no sound, there was: Pain. It ricocheted down that line and burnt through my heart, smarting my eyes and choking my voice – and someone said, "Shall I call back later?" It might have been me. I put down the cold, black, greasy receiver and the coins rattled down into the box. And I knew.

It was moments later and it was forever that I saw her. Mummy, that is. At the end of the corridor she stood, thrice fractured by the multi-paned glass safety doors that studded its length. It was Mummy. Only that day she was the Angel of Death.

They found her under a tree in the woods – a man and his two dogs out walking early, her barely beating heart still full of pain, despite the stomach full of painkillers that had rendered her cold and unconscious many hours before, and the empty bottle that kept its lonely vigil by her side.

As Mummy's eyes met mine down that long weary corridor she knew that I knew. And the howl that cut through the silence that morning came from nowhere on this earth – and I will hear it for all eternity.

And God asked me to live for us both. And, through tears that I thought would never stop flowing, I made them my promise and sometimes, when the sun is high in the sky and life is so good that my spirit is flying, I am sure that I can hear Sally laughing…

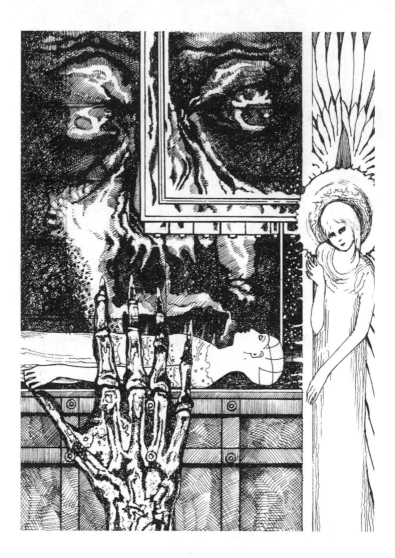

"Between Angels and Demons"

Chapter Thirty One
The Final Day

Christmas is always over too fast.

Usually it sort of drifts on for a little while in a lazy haze of cold turkey sandwiches, mince pies, small scraps of wrapping paper peeking out from underneath armchairs and bizarre confectionery (commonly involving ginger) that only ever appears at Christmas. Fuelled by my relentless enthusiasm for celebrations and stoked by Jeremy's birthday on the 27th December, Christmas in our house tended to last longer than most but still it was always over too fast.

This year, however, it was even more critical that Christmas did not end. Because this year there was nothing on the other side. December 27th was the date they had given me for the start of my radiotherapy treatment. So that was the day that must never come. So Jeremy would never have his birthday, but Christmas would last forever and so he wouldn't mind so much.

At least that was how I saw it.

But Time does keep marching. However hard you wrest and struggle with him with your will, however hard you entreat him to pause and rest a while – or sometimes, even, forever – in a moment of your choosing, he marches sternly on, gaze fixed to the fore, footsteps tireless as the day the world began. And so he barely noticed me, tugging urgently at his sleeve, as he strode on by towards the Final Day. Instead he left me there by the wayside; to cry myself to sleep - and to be borne inexorably into another day…

And, indeed, the day did come. The sun did rise and Fate won our feisty battle to see me on the road to the Churchill Hospital in Oxford for my first session of radiotherapy.

So here I was in Oxford after all: such a strange and painful irony. Far from my mystical 'dreaming spires', the hospital that loomed before us was drab and grey, cold and forbidding. And I was here not to stimulate and celebrate my young and eager mind but to have that brain blasted with potentially lethal levels of radiation in the hope of eradicating a sly and evil foe that snaked a deadly path within.

As we crossed the threshold into the building, we crossed once more into the 'other' world. The dark, dank corridors, with their peeling walls and dripping ceilings, drew us, Mummy and me, hungrily down into their black, dis-topian lair, ever nearer to its fearful core. With each step, urgent and furious, I built my wall back up around me, rueing the day that I had, so irresponsibly, let it down. And then we had arrived and somehow a warm and smiling lady doctor had also found herself in this alien and hostile world. And she knew my name and sat us down and told me not to be afraid. But I was.

And then she looked sad and told me that I would have to brace myself for some difficult news. The treatment was going to cause me to lose all my beautiful hair. And I reached up to my black felt hat and flowing golden cascade and whipped them smartly off my head. "I already did," I grinned, and we laughed. How we all laughed. And suddenly the light shone in on this dark underworld and, in that moment, I knew that however high my wall stood, God would always find me.

The monster was terrifying. Huge and black and cold it filled the spartan concrete room from end to end; a vast mechanical predator squatting in its barren, hostile lair.

On one wall, utterly incongruous, was a poorly painted mural – a crass, lurid depiction of an idealised landscape that, contrary to intentions, served only to emphasise the hard, industrial chill that pervaded the room.

And they had not led me to sacrifice unadorned. The florid purple markings that segmented my soft, naked scalp bound me inescapably in to the nightmare realm, preparing my soft, naked brain to be offered up to the mercy of the beast. But it wouldn't see my fear.

So I climbed up to the sacrificial stone and stretched out along its length. And then they took over my body as well as my soul and moved and contorted it to their desired position until they were satisfied. And afterwards they ran, all of them, to hide, out of sight of the beast's fatal glare, behind the safety of their fortress-thick walls and space-age clothing. And they left me. And they told me that if I moved, even the tiniest fraction, the beast would take my thoughts, my intellect, my emotions and my capacity to live and burn them out of me forever. And so I screwed up everything very tight within me and kept still. And because I held on to him so tightly Fear stayed very quiet and still too - and the beast might not have noticed the little, involuntary twitches and jerks that he really couldn't help but give. We hoped not.

And so each day, as the Three Wise Men journeyed towards Epiphany and beyond, I journeyed towards hell and back: fourteen days that are really forever. And at the end of my journey, instead of the Christ child wrapped in swaddling clothes and lying in a manger, I saw a little girl. Her drugged and lifeless form lay weightily in her father's arms. Her bald, graffitied head lolled moronically to one side as, against every natural instinct, he carried her past me down the corridor, compelled inexorably into the lair. Then, just for a moment, he stopped and he drew that limp fragile doll so tightly to himself that I thought my heart might break as well as his, and I didn't need to see his tears to know that sometimes the world goes mad and, lost and alone, all you can do is stumble blindly in the dark and pray that if your soul cries out loudly enough The Good Shepherd knows where to find you...

149

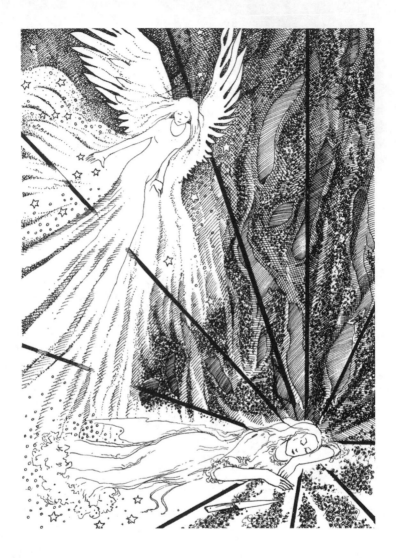

""It isn't me!""

Chapter Thirty Two
Mad, Bad and Dangerous to Know

Even I, with my capacious capacity for optimism, have to admit that January is, at the best of times, a gloomy month. This year it was positively interminable. Two weeks of cranial radiotherapy had not been altogether my preferred way to see in the New Year and with all the glittery distractions of Christmas well and truly 'wrapped up' there was little on the horizon to gladden a thoroughly 'cheesed off' heart. The truth was that I was bored – even the Shepherd's Pie was beginning to pall – and I was becoming aware that the hardest part of having a 'terminal illness' might actually be the small, quiet hours rather then the acute moments of melodrama that one is carried through on the waves of crisis. Adjusting to being at home was at the same time wonderful and difficult for all concerned. The mountain of medication to be choreographed in to an average day was overwhelming. This feeling was compounded – albeit not without mirth – by Daddy's mind-boggling 'medication made simple' chart, and to add insult to injury I had on my first day home suffered a near-death experience at the hands of one particularly large tablet that had become inadvertently lodged in my windpipe.

More insidious (if less dramatic!) were the longer-term effects of those drugs that were gradually making themselves more apparent as the weeks passed. For the doctors, it was the impact of the medication on the rogue cancer cells that was of interest; what was the odd loss of feeling in the finger-tips, the "possibly permanent" nervous tick in the face or the rapid degeneration of the eyesight, provided the leukaemia was under control? For me, and for my family, though, the equation was not such a simple one. Of course the control of the cancer was of paramount importance but it did not stop the increasing trade-off for that control being alien and frightening.

The pain seeped into every fibre of my being, drawing attention to muscles and nerves that I had never even known I had. Even the tiny muscles behind my eyes, my cheekbones and my jaw screamed their protest night and day, cursing any attempts to raise up out of bed to take a bath or dress myself. Defiantly I braved their wrath to climb shakily down the little wooden staircase from my room and lie for a while in the small cosy sitting room beside the kitchen - but there was always a cost to such reckless abandon.

The pain, however, I could bear. The exhaustion, I told myself, was my body's way of curbing my impatient spirit whilst it set about making me strong once more. No, it was the madness that nearly got me…

It crept stealthily across my mind; so soft and fleet of foot that I can't really tell you when it first came to roost. For a long time we thought that it was me - thought that Terror had finally won out over my determined but exhausted spirit - and those months were the worst. We looked on, helpless, my family and I, and I could feel it slipping away and knew that I was losing my mind. Sometimes it was in the little things that we could see it, irrational fears, even hallucinations, that gripped and strangled my sense of reason and reality, but at others it was more assertive, exploding its way into our hitherto mild and sunny world with a violence and anger that tore up the ground from beneath our feet.

It was, for the demons, the ultimate triumph. And how they revelled in this, their finest hour. Like the proverbial parasite, they had wormed their way to the very core of my being, overwhelming resistance and weakening defences to possess not merely my body but the spirit too, the very thing that made me. It was with a shocking and remorseless glee that they set about utilising their newly occupied stronghold.

"It isn't me!" I heard myself scream as the demons picked up and hurled anything they could get their hands on at the people I loved more than life itself. "It isn't me," I whimpered, exhausted and afraid as I lay semi-conscious on the cold stone floor, having been unable to resist the demons' lure to bang my head repeatedly and rhythmically against the wall. "It isn't me," I pleaded with Jeremy to understand, as I chased him maniacally around the house with a knife in my hand, the demons in my head and terror in my heart. "It isn't me."

And it wasn't. I could feel them when they were looming, black and vile, warping and defiling my rose-tinted view of the world so that I saw out of their eyes instead of mine. Waking or asleep I could hear them, tormenting and goading me, persuading me to accept their will and consign my own to oblivion. I saw them in the mirror when I washed, smelt them on my breath and on my skin and could feel them straining at the confines of my skull till I feared it would split and crack with the force of their evil. And then, all of a sudden, they would leave; disappear without a word and leave us all trembling, wondering if they had gone forever or if they would be back again once more to leave carnage in their wake and despair on the wind…

And they always were back. Just when we had begun to trust again, they came. And each time it was the same until, one day, when the Demons summoned up all their strength and threw a chair at her retreating back, Mummy couldn't bear it any more. And instead of telling them she told me, and I had never felt so lost and alone. And nor had she. And she telephoned my doctors and said that I would have to live in the hospital, because she couldn't cope any more. And we cried and I pleaded and held on to her and told her that I wouldn't let them win next time – but we both knew that it wasn't up to me.

So we sat there together, Mummy and I, in front of the doctors, and laid our souls bare on the cheap, laminate-top desk. And the doctors dissected them thoroughly and made scribbled notes and murmured comments. And then they told us that they couldn't help us and so we picked up the torn and ragged remnants of our souls and draped them as best we could about our shoulders and turned softly on our heels to leave. And perhaps something touched them in the way that we did so, for they called us back and offered us a parting gift of hope.
 The psychiatrist, they said, was experienced in cases like mine – if we liked they would arrange a meeting... Psychiatry, I'd often thought, must be a fascinating discipline. I had even considered, in that strangely abstract, ill-informed sort of way that one ponders one's future career when one is confronted with a list of A-Level options, studying for a future as a psychiatrist, only to be dissuaded on discovering that I would have to take a science qualification in the place of Fine Art. Thus the idea took its place on my 'virtual' shelf of reserve careers, right next to show-jumper and to the far left of prima-ballerina, actress, opera-singer, and pop-star, all of which were absolutely perfect, aside for, in each case, one minor detail (eg. no horse or the fact that I gave up ballet lessons at age 8). Nevertheless the concept still fascinated me, and the older I became the more conscious I was of the

subtlety and complexity behind our day-to-day actions and decisions; the unspoken, and very often unrecognised, motivation that governs our entire behaviour. Observing the phenomenon in those around me, however, was one thing. To be lain out upon the Couch of Revelation myself was another matter entirely. If I had hidden motivations behind my behaviour then I trusted that they were hidden for a very good reason, thank you very much, and it would be much the best thing to leave them that way. Still, I had to confess that this current run of psychopathic mania had to stop, and if this fellow might bring me one step closer to that end then it was surely worth a try.

And so there I was that Monday morning, bolt upright in a very un-couch-like NHS chair, and 100% prepared to give absolutely nothing away: a constructive start. He sat, equally upright, opposite me, the whole room carrying a distinctly 'Inquisition-type' air about it, and we waited. I wasn't quite sure what we were waiting for, but since I knew that I had absolutely nothing to say, the onus, I felt, was on him to start the ball rolling. After a not insignificant while spent in this tranquil repose, however, I began to suspect that he, in fact, felt the metaphorical ball to be in my court. It really was all rather like a game. A kind of 'who can hold out the longest' game where the competitors, (this was definitely the competitive type of game), stare at each other unblinking until one or other 'breaks'. Well, I have always had a competitive streak, but frankly his chances were not helped by the fact that I really did not have a clue what I was supposed to say. So there we sat and we might be still there to this day were it not for the fact that I suddenly recalled Mummy's scared, exhausted face as she righted the chair that I had aimed so violently at her loving, benevolent retreating form. And I knew that I was never going to let that happen again.

I smiled tentatively and began to speak…

To learn that it was my medication that was responsible for my madness was both an unbearable irony and an enormous relief. 'Steroid Psychosis', my psychiatrist diagnosed shortly into our meetings, reassuring us that when I stopped taking the tablets the 'side effects' would cease. The fact that I had another two years worth of the shiny red pills to take was definitely a minus, but the joy in realising that the terrifying change in my personality was down to a temporary invasion was immense. The demons were fed-up, but for Mummy the news meant a chance to gather up once more the last vestige of her morale and keep holding on. For me, the knowledge that I was not in fact losing my marbles opened up once more the glorious horizon that lay beyond these years of treatment and marked the beginning of the rest of my life… And until then it gave me back the spirit and the strength to fight another day and the faith to know that when I finally stepped out into that fresh new dawn it would be as myself – a little stronger and perhaps a little wiser – but I would still be me.

So put that in your pipe and smoke it, Demons…

Chapter Thirty Three
'Bizarre/Good'

Still, all that was the wrong kind of excitement and if, on reflection, zooming back in to that endless afternoon in January, whilst I concede that I was not exactly bored, I was nevertheless decidedly fed up and seriously considering joining the Foreign Legion, when I remembered the phone number. Though scrawled haphazardly on a seemingly unassuming scrap of paper, the number was clearly worth considerably more than its weight in gold if the sense of ceremony and 'cat that got the cream'ishness with which it was purveyed to my hospital bedside that morning had been anything to go by. If God had had his own hot- line to heaven, the number could not have been borne with greater reverence, so I was not altogether surprised at the quivering revelation that this was in fact Jimmy Saville's private number that he had expressly requested be passed on to me. Still, the idea of actually calling said number definitely fell into one of my 'bizarre' categories and, even after our bedside 'tete a tetes', I couldn't quite picture the way a 'hi! Just called up for a chat!' kind of conversation might go. Consequently, despite a faint but nagging temptation in all those 'un-fixed' dreams just itching to be fulfilled – though admittedly at this point how much I still longed to hose down elephants with Johnny Morris required some consideration – I had, until now, pretty much put the number out of my mind.

Nevertheless, desperate times called for desperate measures and it's surprising what desperation can do for a little social awkwardness. In fact, frankly, it was astonishing. Not 100% convinced that he would even register who I was when I called, the overwhelming warmth of the esteemed 'Fixer of Dreams', 'Fulfiller of Wishes', on hearing my voice, all but singed my eyebrows in its intensity. He had, it seemed, been awaiting my call and was most offended that I had been so long about it. Well, what do you know?

Anyway with social niceties out of the way – and when I had picked myself up off the floor – we got down to business. He had, he said, a job for me at the hospital and, if I were well enough, would I help out? Now it is a strange and wonderful thing about being struck down by a particularly dire kind of illness but one is suddenly aware of just how fortunate one is. Not only that but, more poignantly, one is also suddenly and acutely conscious of how much less fortunate the lives of others can be. For me, this dual realisation had early on given rise to a passionate desire to 'make a difference', to 'give back' for the privilege of being alive and if Jim thought that there was some small way in which I could help then I was there. Mysteriously, he would tell me little more about my brief than the time and date of our assignation and by the end of our call I was feeling decidedly James Bond-ish about the task in hand and altogether more excited about life… And, after all, the Foreign Legion would never have appreciated all that I had to offer…

(Plus, I've heard they have peas under their mattresses…)

Chapter Thirty Four
Surprise!

Zero hour was to be ten o'clock on a fine Monday morning; the meeting place, the Spinal Injuries Centre, Stoke Mandeville Hospital. There was, Jim had said, someone he wanted to introduce me to before the mission got underway.

And so, bright and early, there I was, and there was Jim. And then, there was Michael.

So far in my lifetime I must have bumped into, brushed past, sidled by – not to mention tripped up – an extraordinary number of people. It has always been a remarkable thing to me that such a tiny percentage of those zillions of fleeting relationships develop into something more lasting and that still fewer have any significant bearing upon one's life. Still more curious, it seems to me, is that these special few might arise out of anywhere and at any time – usually, in my experience, when and where one least expects it. Well, Michael, I feel privileged to say, was destined to become one of those special few and, looking back, I think that from that very first moment when we said hello, my life was already changed forever...

Dr. Michael Rogers is 'disabled'. And yet he is one of the most 'able' people I have ever known. How strange is our conditioned perception of the world; how strange, and how blind. But then I could perhaps have dipped into the wisdoms of the School of Political Correctness and failed to mention, or even to notice, the fact that since contracting a freak virus at the age of twenty-three,

Michael has been unable to move any part of his body from the neck down. I could refrain from drawing attention to the wheelchair that he controls with his chin and has over the past forty years become an extension of himself. I could smile and pretend and tell you that to all intents and purposes the physical restrictions on Michael's life are an irrelevance.

But they're not, and in so doing, it seems to me, I would be 'failing to mention', 'refraining from drawing attention to', positively ignoring everything that is most 'able', everything that is extraordinary, about him, and what it was that was impressed upon my spirit on that very first day and has been a guiding influence in my life ever since.

To know Michael was, increasingly, to alter my perception of the human spirit forever. What I fought was a battle with death. What Michael had, it seemed to me, fought and won was a battle with life. My fight was intense and finite – live or die – Michael's was a long, drawn-out wrestling with those inner demons, the ultimate test of the spirit. Two years after leaving the army, fate had thrown down the gauntlet and he would spend his life rising to that challenge; each day that he woke up and smiled he would conquer the enemy, only to face him again the next morning, sword in hand.

And yet, paradoxically, there is a profound peace about him: not a placid, quiet peace but a lively, animated one, as if in a lifetime of learning he has found a place of acceptance of his condition without being 'resigned' to it. His world is one not of thwarted hopes and long-abandoned dreams but one of progress and creativity. For every channel blocked by Fate, Courage and Determination cut two more, forging through hitherto uncharted territory. Were it not for the fact that, one terrible day nearly half a century ago, a young man was struck down by a crippling virus that paralysed his body and released his mind, the field of research into spinal injuries would be gravely the poorer and at least one young woman may not have found the inspiration to take up Fate's challenge with a whoop and a cry and a triumphant anticipation of the new roads that lay ahead...

Still, more of that later. For now, the clock is ticking. It's Zero Hour plus one and the mission briefing is underway...

I was, it seemed, to be deputy to Michael's 'Big Cheese' – he had the clipboard – and the idea was to surprise a young paraplegic woman who lived in the hospital's 'halfway house' and had just, against all odds, given birth to a healthy little girl. Now I could well appreciate what a wonderful, miraculous thing this was, but exactly how we were to surprise her no one had actually thought to mention to me. Were we perhaps to leap out of a cupboard as she, blissfully unaware, passed merrily by? Did the plan involve inflated balloons and strategically wielded drawing pins? Even "Boo!" when declaimed with adequate zeal can have, in my experience, a remarkably satisfactory result on a hitherto relaxed subject...

Well, at this rate, I was liable to be as surprised as she was about the whole affair when it actually happened. And then - just as I was thinking that very thought - it did and I was.

There we were, Michael and I, sitting, blissfully unaware (well, at least one of us was), talking over strategy whilst failing to get to the hub of the matter, when in walked the Duchess of York. Now this must be what's known as true 'fame'; to be able to walk into a room without so much as a poorly executed 'Boo' – or even a polite sneeze

– and to give anyone who happened to be in there the biggest surprise they ever had in their lives! Imagine..! I wonder whether the novelty wears off after a time or rather that it becomes increasingly satisfying? What might the effect be if such a person were to combine their initial advantage with an animated leap out of a wardrobe when one was least expecting it? Hmmm – no end of possibilities...

Anyway, where was I? Ah yes – well and truly surprised. And, since Michael seemed a good deal less so, I surmised that the arrival was not altogether unexpected and that this might well be the nature of the surprise that awaited the young woman that we were, I presumed, still waiting for. And so it was.

And the Duchess liked the joke and I liked her and we all laughed a lot and became friends. And somewhere along the way I remembered that, though the world may be full of surprises, they don't all leave one fighting for one's life – and very often they just make one smile...

Chapter Thirty Five
The Three Musketeers

It was the 'small print' in my next big mission brief that really had me intrigued. "Wear 'something smart'", Jim had said as he filled me in on the usual 'specs'; time, date and location. Since his idea of 'smart' tended towards favouring a gold-lame tracksuit as opposed to a regular gold nylon one, I wasn't altogether confident that I had anything in my wardrobe to fit the bill, but I decided to go with my own interpretation on the theme ('smart', that is, rather then gold lame) and hoped it would suffice.

Thus, at 9am on the dot, I arrived at the Spinal Injuries Centre, sporting a chic little baby-blue suit and hoping that if I wasn't exactly doing 'glitz' I might be doing 'elegance' instead. Jim was sporting an even broader smile than usual, which was bordering on the disconcerting, but, as I followed his grinning form through the maze of outbuildings and lawns behind the hospital wing, the faint flutter of butterflies in my tummy were, I knew, more down to excitement than nerves. How misguided one can be!

Our destination, when we arrived, could not have been more apparent. In a roundabout way we had found ourselves at the hospital's giant sports stadium and race track and, by the looks of things – and via a more direct route - so had an increasing number of other people who were busy settling themselves into the vast ribbons of seating that encircled the field. Jim led me to a small row of individual chairs at the edge of the track and sat me down.

"Wait here," he instructed, "I'll be back in a minute," and before I knew it he'd vanished into the gathering throng.

It was a glorious sunny morning and the magnificent stadium had on its proudest face as it glowed and preened in the beneficent, golden light. More than absorbed by the scene and the growing activity around me, I barely noticed the next half hour as it passed and went and it wasn't until the other four seats beside me filled up and Jim had still not appeared that I started to wonder where he was. I still had no idea what I was required to do, and by the look of things I was about to be doing it nevertheless! Still, I was distracted for a moment by a smiley-faced woman who handed me a very official looking programme, the cover of which announced proudly that I was about to attend the World Wheelchair Olympic Games.

Well, this was all terribly exciting and at least I now knew what we were all here for, but I was still none the wiser as to how I could help out. Should I not, at this very moment perhaps, be handing out programmes or seeing people to seats? I glanced around, this time more anxiously, for Jim but to no avail. Once again I distracted myself with the programme and it was then that I saw it. 'Visiting Dignitaries', the first page heading ran, followed by a short and important looking list of five names. The first four were undoubtedly very impressive, consisting as they did of various presidents of countries and Olympic organisations but it was the fifth name on this highly prestigious list that really caused my jaw to drop. In bold, black, indelible type there it was;

Miss Emma Bowes – Friend of the Duchess of York.

I had barely had time to retrieve my jaw from my lap,

accompanied lustily by the jubilant brass band, when it became clear that my first duty – whatever that might be - was about to be fulfilled. The smiley lady was back, this time to usher her five important charges to their feet and – it became apparent – towards the centre of the stadium! Wearing what I hoped was my own most winning and confident smile, I followed my leader out on to the track. Feeling more and more like a confidence trickster as each moment went by, I took my place obediently at the end of the line, speculating inwardly how long it would be before I was, extremely publicly, rumbled and wondering what, in the meantime I might be expected to do. Just as I was entertaining the rather alarming thought that I might be required to 'perform' in some way – why oh why had I ever told Jim about my aspirations for the stage? – I was blessedly distracted by the arrival of a very noisy helicopter.

My relief on seeing the Duchess of York step elegantly out of said vehicle was twofold. Crucially, the limelight had, in an instant, shifted very firmly from myself and from my dignified friends to the real star of the show, but it was also, and the irony was not lost on me here, a profound relief to see a familiar face. As she ambled politely down the line, shaking hands and enquiring after health, I tried to look as much like I had expected to be there as possible whilst at the same time wondering what on earth she was going to do when she saw me, the fraudster, loitering shamelessly at the end of the row.

And then she laughed. And all of a sudden it didn't matter where we were or who was watching, because I had never felt more at ease. We laughed and laughed and once again she liked the joke and I liked her – immensely. And the cameras clicked and whirred and we laughed some more and said goodbye and I didn't feel like a fraudster any more – because I really was a friend of the Duchess of York and something told me I always would be…

So there we were, me, Jim and Michael – as bizarre a take on the Three Musketeers as you are ever likely to seek – and 'Boy!' did we have some adventures! Sometimes it was just me and Michael and sometimes just me and Jim – and just occasionally the Duchess was there too! – but it was always extraordinary. With Michael I learnt that nothing is impossible – and if you can't paint with your hands then you could always try with your mouth. With Jim I learnt that you never know what life might spring upon you at any time, so it's best to expect anything and hold on to your hat!

And above all I learnt that no matter how fiendish the demon's dance, no matter how dark the night-time shadows, life was still out there for the living, and I meant to take its outstretched hand and dance to the horizon and beyond – and never look back…

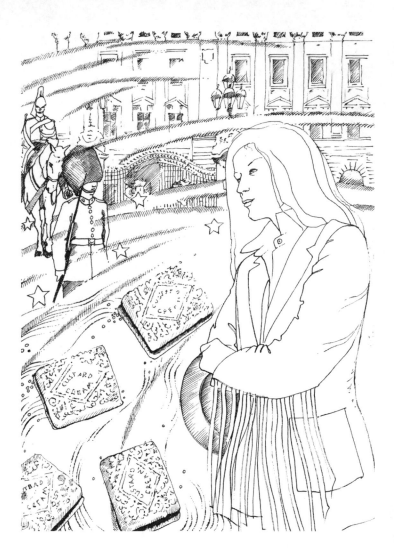

"Moments later our magic carpet pulled up outside the
Palace door..."

Chapter Thirty Six
The Princess and
the Tea

If there's one thing Jim is good at, it's surprises. But, as
you've seen, his aren't the leaping out of a wardrobe
shouting "Boo!" kind of surprises, the kind that make
you jump out of your skin. His are the kind that make
you wonder if you have jumped out of the real world
altogether.

This is the story of the day I went to Buckingham Palace
for tea.

Actually, the first time I went to Buckingham Palace for
tea I was with Jeremy. I was five years old and he was
three. The Queen was in that day, Daddy told us, as the
flag was flying. "Good," said Jeremy, "shall we go in
for tea?" But we had to go and catch our train so there
wasn't time to keep our engagement. Still, we did get an
ice-cream instead. And she would have all the biscuits
herself, so we thought she wouldn't mind too much.

Well this time I was in a taxi and instead of Jeremy I was
with Jim. Which was already quite surprising now I think
about it. He had to call on a friend of his and he wondered
if I would mind hanging around for a while whilst they
caught up with some business. It wasn't as if I had
anything particularly pressing to attend to so I smiled
agreeably and settled back to watch the London world
go by. I loved London. I loved the vibrancy, the energy,
the Life that teemed along every street, that gathered on
every corner. And above all, perhaps, I loved the

Possibility. London was a place where anything could happen.

And it was just about to.

As always, as we swung round the Big Corner and into The Mall I had the sense that I was swinging out of the everyday world and into Storybook London. Even without the mounted guards and the gilded iron railings somehow this part of town belonged more to Christopher Robin and the elusive Alice than it did to the throngs of day-trippers who lounged untidily about the steps of the monument, sporting state-of-the-art cameras, rucksacks and dubious souvenir flags. How strange, I thought, to be Her Majesty and know that every time you peeped out of your bedroom window you would be greeted by hoards of strangers waving those dubious flags and speculating as to whether you were at home!

Still, I couldn't resist a sideways glance at the Palace as it swung into view. Perhaps if I had been looking at Jim instead I'd have noticed his grin. "Just pull in here, driver," he chuckled. And I chuckled too.

But then we did! Just like that we drew up at those big, black Storybook gates, smiled winningly at the Storybook guards and we were inside! Moments later our magic carpet pulled up outside the Palace door. I waved at Christoper Robin and in we went.

Well, who'd have thought the Queen was a fan of 'Jim'll Fix It'? Perhaps she'd written asking for him to remove all those flag-waving strangers for the day. It certainly explained why he'd always been too busy to answer my letters.

The footmen were, of course, immensely courteous as

they showed us into the lift. Far more so, I would suggest, than was due to such a shady pair as we. Had I had some inkling that I might have been spending the afternoon in the company of royalty I would undoubtedly have thought twice about my relaxed ensemble of suede cowboy jacket and jeans. My grandmother would despair of me, though to be frank, she would have despaired even more of Jim, who seemed to have a tracksuit for all occasions. Queen Victoria, I felt, would not have been amused as we clambered inelegantly into her lift, reputedly her favourite room (yes, indeed, 'room') in the house. Surveying our surroundings as we rose, I was inclined to believe the rumours. Its plush, ornate interior seemed more to invite an afternoon's rest and repose than a transitory visit between floors.

Then we were taking softly cushioned footsteps along the upstairs corridor, sunlight pouring in through the windows. And in its white-gold silence we were a thousand miles, a hundred years, from the roaring immediacy of the world without the gates.

The Duchess met us at the door. Her smile was warm and amused as she ushered us in to her relaxed, unpretentious apartment. Our visit was clearly less of a surprise to her than it was to me! Moments later we were sitting squashily on the sofa, a plate of custard creams between us and freshly made tea on the long low table. Pleasantries were exchanged merrily; "How lovely to see you again"; "Do help yourself to custard creams", "If it is too warm in here do feel free to remove your hair" – you know the kind of thing. And whilst I sat there, bald and happy, doing more than justice – on Jeremy's behalf – to the biscuits, she and Jim got down to business.

When it was time to put on our hats, coats and hair once again, the Duchess grinned impishly and dashed out of the room. Preceded momentarily by an infectious bubbling laugh she bounded back into the room, triumphantly sporting a fine head of platinum blonde hair that Marilyn Monroe would have been proud to call her own. "Blondes, after all," she said, "notoriously had more fun," and certainly the wig had caused a great deal of merriment one evening with friends! But, the Duchess felt, it would suit me far better than it had suited her, and just to prove it she fetched a mirror and straightened my new hair atop my head.

A few minutes later, as we climbed back into our waiting cab I smiled contentedly to myself. After all it's not every day you go to tea with a Princess and it's surely even less often that you come away wearing her hair.

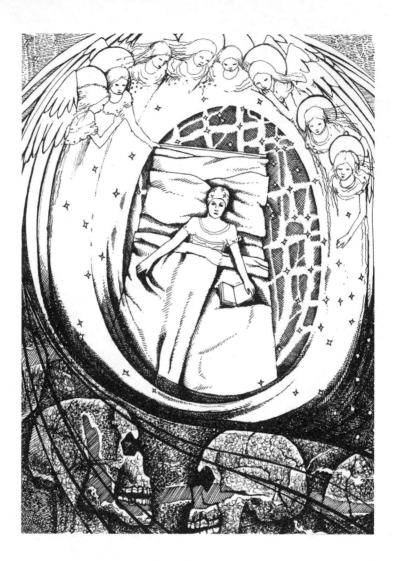

"And we all knew who was winning..."

Chapter Thirty Seven
Back into the Fray

The Demons, though, had not entirely lost their sting. Undoubtedly, as the months passed and my daily trips for intravenous chemo became routine, the dozens of pills that lined the back of the little pine table in the kitchen slipped down more easily and my hair even started to grow back, so the memory of their spite, once burnt so blackly on my soul, began to fade. Like Technicolor photographs in a weary sheet of monochrome newsprint, my extraordinary adventures illuminated the day-to-day trial of 'maintenance' chemotherapy, providing respite from its chilling, grey monotony. My days were filled with light and colour that drew attention away from the shadows and gave my dazed and weary sprit harbour from the storm. But the sky always carried a threat; the clouds were gathering on the horizon and I knew now how to read the signs…

The doctors had decided that another 'intensification block' would be prudent, just to let the demons know that we hadn't forgotten they were out there. The block was 'booked-in' for May, four weeks before my re-scheduled interview for Oxford and in good time to ensure that I would be well and truly bald once again in time for the occasion…

Going back into the arena again, my wounds still raw from the last battle, was against every instinct I had ever had. If the last fight had almost killed me how was I to survive a fresh onslaught in my now desperately weakened state, with neither the artillery of health nor the armour of ignorance? Still, I trusted them, my doctors, who had

had to watch and pray with us for more than six months now and know that, whilst it was thanks to them that I was still alive, it was also their decisions that fuelled each anguished spate of vomiting, prompted each contorted twist of pain, and I knew that they would not put my thin, ravaged body through more than they felt absolutely necessary.

And so there I was once again, back in my little room and setting up the barricade. Three of my most stalwart teddy-bear friends, a clutch of photographs and a fighting spirit may not seem much against the might of the demons, but it was what they represented – the love and security that had carried me not only through the past terrifying months but over nineteen years of scraped knees, bruised egos and broken hearts – that gave them their power.

And this time, at least, we were ready for them…

In reality, knowing the ropes may have made things less alien, but observing my body in its rapid and agonising decline once more was no less horrific. The drugs took their time in working on the new, soft, pioneering strands of hair that capped my head, but, even as I watched, the rest of the ground that I had tended and nurtured over the past few months' respite simply crumbled away. Content with nothing less than my entire body and soul, the demons revelled in their victory, taunting and mocking as I was forced to abandon my dignity along with my strength, in complete acquiescence to my newly incapacitated state and 'the system'. Lying there drugged and confused, they taunted, and in this continual semi-stupor, how could the hallowed halls of Oxford have ever been for me anything but an impossible dream? And they cackled and patted each other on the back for hitting out just where it hurt most.

But if they thought I was going to give them that satisfaction then they had never been more wrong. They forgot that this time I had experienced the miracle of regeneration. I knew that my poor assailed body, though tired and weakened from the fray, would, at every possible moment of relief, turn and rally its troops for the counter response. Even as it reeled from the last blow, it would be gathering its resources within and re-forming its campaign.

I had observed the astonishing healing of my chemically bludgeoned arm, watching wide-eyed as, against all the expectations of the doctors, the swelling subsided and the huge weeping sore began to close. I had seen the new, perfect skin drawing across the abyss, almost before my eyes, until the hideous deformity was just a memory, as if 'magic-ed' away with the shimmering touch of a wand or kissed better by the tender lips of a passing angel...

I knew, then, that my body was a continuous miracle and that while there was life there really was hope. And I sensed too that, whilst it got on with the task at the 'nuts and bolts' level, just as crucial was my role in maintaining my spirit; my conviction that I would win through. And so I mocked the demons right back, poked out my tongue and told them that time would tell which of us was the wiser but that I had the angels on my side so, for them, the odds did not look good. And I saw them quake a little and retreat a little further from the foot of my bed. And, looking them directly in the eyes, I reached out and took a book, Wuthering Heights, from my nightstand, opened it at Chapter One and began to read...

And we all knew who was winning...

Chapter Thirty Eight
A Rolling Stone

At the time I had thought it a coincidence, but in retrospect I'm not so sure that it wasn't a very calculated choreography on Mummy's part. Anyway, however it came about, I was all set to spend the week before my Oxford interviews – yes, plural, one with each of my prospective tutors and one with the Principal of the college – with some absolutely lovely friends of the family in whose company we had all had some magical and very laid-back times in the past. God lived in their house too and memorable associations were rife; of horse riding through the Herefordshire countryside; Mars Bars in the basement 'Dive'; home made banana-splits in the dining room – not to mention some very rowdy, and not altogether honourable, games of something that might almost pass as water-polo in the indoor pool. Suffice to say that, though I had not stayed with them alone before, the invitation had been a sunny, happy window to look to just beyond this latest bout in hospital, and I was looking forward to seeing everyone again.

The expedition was not without some trepidation, however. 'Everyone' included their children, a boy and their four girls, the youngest of whom was only three, and the last time I had seen them all I was fit, tanned and bounding with energy. How would they respond to my frail, emaciated form, not to mention my increasingly naked scalp?

Yes, as expected, once again my hair was beginning to fall. This time the soft, short strands seemed simply to 'wear away' in patches – perhaps as they rubbed against my pillow – resulting in a tortuous 'moth-eaten' effect that disturbed my already long-traumatised mind beyond bearing. In the end it was not so much the 'falling' as the waiting that drove me crazy. Each morning as, once again, I woke choking on the feathery strands, it was the horror of the past six months, the terror of the known and of what was yet to come that caught in my throat and stuffed up my nostrils so that I could barely breathe.

And so I pulled it all out.

One terrible morning Daddy awoke to find me standing barefoot on the lawn, my flimsy nightdress teased by the early summer breeze as the morning sun cast its shadows into the new day. But I didn't see him. I didn't see the sunshine, the shadows, or the new-green leaves that danced on that playful breeze. I saw only the blackness inside and knew only that I couldn't wait any more. And I reached up and tore at my scalp, tore out in handfuls the soft baby-blond that clung tickling to my warm tears as it fell. And I didn't stop until every last strand was freed and the waiting was over and I could turn and cry into Daddy's arms...

So the Demons and I continued our merry dance. And some days they led and, others I, but deep down I sensed that they no longer wrote the tune. And it is a strange phenomenon, but one day you wake up and find that at some point along the way the alien horrors that at first paralysed your mind to its very core have sidled in to your everyday routine. You realise that life does go on beyond the end of the world and it carries you rolling, for better or worse, along with it. Well, whilst I was still along for the ride, one thing was for sure, I was not going to let the moss have even a moment to gather..!

Indeed my holiday galloped by, in a thunder of hooves and the chattering of happy voices, and I even entrusted my naked head to the love and compassion that enveloped me from the moment I arrived. And all too soon it was time to go home and goodbyes were ringing out across the Malvern Hills and promises were being made to "Write soon!" and "Come again!"

Then I settled back into my seat, warm and content, peaceful and relaxed...! But yikes! Of course! 'Going home' was not the entire story. In fact at that moment it by no means merited even a mention in the footnotes. We had a stop-off to make on the way – and it wasn't just for sandwiches...

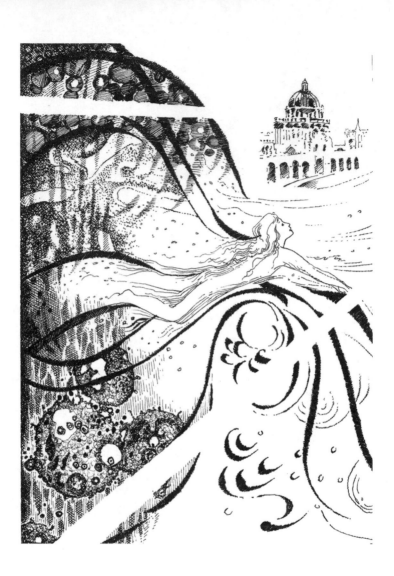

""Anything is possible...believe...believe...""

Chapter Thirty Nine
The Promised Land

As Oxford's dreaming spires rose into view, the full extent of my mother's cunning in arranging for me to be out of the house for the two weeks leading up to my University interviews became stomach-churningly apparent Instead of spending the days tearing out everyone else's hair – for want of my own resource – and ruing all those hours spent watching 'Dynasty' and 'The Cosby Show' when I could have been familiarising myself with the entire canon of English Literature circa. 900 – 1950AD or cultivating impressive hobbies like archaeology or brain surgery – or something… Anyway, INSTEAD of doing that, I (and my long suffering parents) had had a blissfully relaxed few days where the only threat to my blood pressure was an extra large portion of clotted cream ice cream, and the impending meetings had barely even crossed my mind. Still, they were now making up for lost time! It's surprising how much 'ruing' one can get down to during a relatively short car journey and I was definitely going for the record. It wasn't that I hadn't been reading over the past few weeks – it was more my choice of material that I was not altogether confident about. Now there was always a chance that Agatha Christie or Enid Blyton were on next year's 1st year English Lit. book list – frankly if it was down to me they'd be a core part of the curriculum – but I had to admit that it was doubtful. Interestingly – though, sadly, for my psychiatrist rather than my potential literature tutors – I had found the intense, traumatic world of 'Wuthering Heights' utterly compelling as it carried me along with it, somehow mirroring the dark, emotional angst of the world in which I had suddenly found myself, and thus this was one book that I had read over the past year that I could be pretty sure they had heard of. Other than that, my hope lay in persuading them that, if they did but know it, 'Five on a Treasure Island' – not to mention 'First Term at Mallory Towers' (educational theme) – provided more than adequate resource for contemplation and literary debate. How hard could that be? After all I had found them resourceful enough to merit innumerable re-readings over the past ten years...

Consoling myself with this rather shaky logic, I turned to the window and determined to focus on the fantastical sandstone cityscape, which by degrees was absorbing me into its 'mellifluous' warmth as we passed along The High and into the heart of the university town. As the outskirts of the town receded I felt them draw to a 'close' behind me, just as the Red Sea did behind the passage of the Israelites, sealing me in to the ancient world of academe where time stood still and even the very stone basked in the reflective glory of wisdom and learning. What could I bring to this auspicious place? Could I really do justice to the honour of being here and the years of guidance and opportunity that had brought me this far? Yes! a part of me sang triumphantly. Yes! And the part of me that is more humble and reserved nodded quietly and qualified my initial response to a passionate surety that, if I were but given the chance, I would give my all to doing so. And like I've said before, I have a lot of all to give...

As we pulled up outside Regents Park College where I was to meet the first of my Inquisitors, I realised with a jolt that the dream had become a reality. From here on it was up to me. As I stood there at the gateway to the college, I stood too at the gateway to the real world. Suddenly their acceptance of me to read English Language and Literature at Oxford University was about much more than a lifetime of dreaming and ambition – it was about living. Here was the gateway in the wall that had separated me from reality for so long; an opening back into the world of the young and the carefree, where life goes on forever and the future is just around the corner... In that strangely reflective moment, I realised too that deep within I had a core of strength, a kind of courage and stability that I had not registered before. In the same moment I knew that it was because of my experience; because of, not despite, the past nine months of life-threatening trauma. It was as if, as a kind of compensation for all that had happened, God had planted something inside me that made me stronger, something that I knew instinctively would never leave me and that would help me to face, not only this challenge, but all that lay on the road ahead with a new and wiser perspective and the knowledge that I had faced the most terrifying of demons and survived.

I took a deep breath. Well, ready or not, here I come..!

Your average demon behind a closed door, however, is not to be underestimated. As I knocked on the deceptively humble looking entrance to the Senior Common Room, nervously straightening my hair, (as one does, only in my case there was the added concern that it might actually fall off altogether if I wasn't careful), and practising my warmest – and most intelligent – smile, he was definitely the one on my mind. Even so, I wasn't altogether prepared for the extraordinary vision that confronted me as, just as my knuckles were preparing for a return rap, the door swung enthusiastically open.

If one were proposing to illustrate a children's book about a brilliant, if not to say precocious, eccentric Oxford professor, then in one's wildest, most inspired dreams one could not have come up with a more perfect model than that standing before me. It is tempting to feel that there is something in the physiology of a true genius that not only dictates that their eyes are distinctly wild and staring but that, in addition, their hair grows outwards and upwards instead of towards the floor like that of your average mortal: Einstein certainly had it, (as, I seem to recall, did 'Doc', Michael J. Fox's 'professorial' and decidedly 'hirsute' mentor in 'Back to the Future' but I don't know if that counts). Anyway, if this fellow's hair was anything to go by, then I was in the presence of immense intellectual stature – and it seemed to be expanding by the moment. The smile that accompanied the astonishing hair, however, was welcoming and wide and, bolstered by this, I followed it obediently into the room. Equally meekly I settled into the chair that was clearly awaiting my arrival and stole a moment to compose all the singular, remarkable features into one – equally extraordinary, I concluded – face.

But before I had time to contemplate the irony that, in such dramatic contrast to my companion, I had not a wisp of hair to call my own, or the opportunity to reflect on any potential implications this might have with regard to my intellectual capacity, Dr Thompson began to speak. Then followed one of the most exhilarating hours of my life…

After all those months confined to a hospital bed, a stint of flying by the seat of my pants was just what the doctor ordered. As I left the SCR that morning, my mind whirling with images, epithets and allusion, my whole being was palpably alive. I could feel it radiating from within; vibrant, excitable, eagerly anticipating the next 'hit' of intellectual stimulation that would maintain this glorious 'high'.

That's not to say that I had altogether distinguished myself in the event. Sadly, Shakespeare was more his thing than Enid Blyton, but – in my defence – I challenge anyone who is, if (determinedly) not six feet under, then, at times, (admittedly) approaching nigh on five, to set about analysing the Bard's life achievements with insight and verve. Frankly, even picking up my immense volume of the Complete Works would have been more than challenging enough for a good day, let alone a bad. My A-Level study of King Lear, however, was a useful reference point, as was my passionate love of the Zefferelli film version of 'Romeo and Juliet' (which William and I could recite word-for word – that is when our mouths weren't too full of M&Ms – and how many six year olds could say that, I wonder? He'll thank me one day…). Anyway, where was I? Ah yes, 'winging it' magnificently – or, at least, hanging in there – and loving every terrifying minute of it. The whole experience, in fact, was very much akin to the proverbial roller-coaster ride in that it almost seemed to be over before I had the chance to register that it had begun – and, in the meantime, I could not have got off even if I had wanted to…

Still - no time to come up with clichéd metaphors; legs quaking and mind buzzing, it was on to my next assignation.

Tripping back down the long, light corridor towards the bursar's office, I had a chance to peep through the leaded panes to the 'quad' beyond. The immaculately mown lawns, bordered cheerily by obedient rows of brightly coloured bedding plants and bestrewn rather more randomly with languid looking students, were distinctly inviting, bathed as they were in the early summer sun. If I closed my eyes tightly enough I could almost transport myself there, hear the slight rustle of pages caught by a passing breeze, smell the sweet green of the sun-warmed grass and share in the companionable hush of minds deep in contemplation and learning. (Or sleep).

But I wasn't there yet and if I was late in meeting up with Dr Mason, the Senior Tutor of the College who was to be my guide and chauffeur – a great privilege – for the duration of my visit, I might never make it, so I drew myself out of my dreams and hurried down to 'The Star'. 'The Star' is not, as one might imagine, the local pub but rather, I had been briefed, a reference to the large star inlaid in the floor at the entrance to the college and a traditional meeting point for students and tutors alike. Here, sure enough, I found Dr Mason – and a more twinkling, amiable looking fellow one is never likely to meet.

Their thoughtfulness in providing me with a guide – not to mention such an esteemed one – had by no means escaped my notice. My second interview was with the tutor in English Language, a fellow of Hertford College and therefore based a little way across town, and they were keen to ensure that I was not exhausted by the trek. Thus, feeling immensely cosseted, I clambered into the car and off we sped. Or rather, 'meandered', as anyone who is familiar with Oxford's one-way systems will sympathise, but at least the leisurely progress allowed for a few minutes of reassuring 'pep-talk' on the way…

The English Language element of the degree course was not, I had to concede, likely to be my strongest point. What I loved was 'creative writing' and, to Daddy's long-suffering despair – an editor and publisher to the marrow in his bones– my approach to grammar, spelling and the like was about as creative as one could get. As far as I was concerned, they were but tools in aiding the conveyance of mood, meaning or narrative and so long as the word was recognisable then who cared whether it was ideally spelt with one or two s's or ought really be rather closer to its estranged partner of the 'infinitive' persuasion? Well the answer was that this fellow, Dr John Kitely, cared – and so much so that he had spent a lifetime thinking and writing about just that. I was more than a little concerned that we might not be on the same wavelength.

Still, as the twinkling Dr Mason bundled me out of the car and the numerous passing bicycles and I danced our merry, weaving dance down the street towards the college entrance, I could hear the whispers on the wind… "Anything is possible…believe…believe…" and I knew that they were right…

Admittedly ten minutes later I wasn't feeling quite so sure. Of course it wasn't that I didn't know what 'irony' was – it was more how to explain it in less than three hundred fumbling words that was foxing me. My Inquisitor's obvious delight in my wriggling discomfort was not altogether helping matters, and I was very much feeling that as anything other than a profound lesson in humility this meeting was failing dismally. Blessedly though, like a cat who toys with a mouse but was never really hungry, he decided to move on and from there on things started to look up. As we delved further into the heart of the subject, to embrace not merely the origins and meaning of language, but its integral relationship to my very perception of the world, without and within, I felt my heart quicken with anticipation. Once again I found myself responding to the challenge, rising to the opportunity to think on my feet and assess on the spot new ideas and concepts. And then I blew it.

It was right at the end of my interview and the conversation was becoming more personable and relaxed. Mr Kitely's acknowledgement of my illness was considerate, even gentle, and he made it clear that it would not stand in the way of my being considered for a place at the college. What he would not stand for, though, he added firmly, was my being a martyr to my health. Instantly my hackles leapt to attention. How dare he suggest that I might use my illness as an excuse to 'get away' with giving less than 100% to such an opportunity? I threw back at him, leaping to my feet. How poorly he had assessed my character if he could imagine my doing so! I accused wildly.

The poor fellow, for the first time since I had entered the room, was clearly under-rehearsed for his response. As he stumbled his way through an explanation of what he had actually meant by his comment – that I must never be afraid of coming to them when my health was a particular problem, rather than pushing myself too hard, (how well, in fact, he had assessed my character) – I felt a decided, and not a little shameful, sinking of the hackles; and with them went my spirits. My misplaced indignation rang in my ears. How could I have been so rude? I was so determined that they should know that were they to offer me a place I would give every bit as much to the privilege as would a student in full health, that I had blown the very opportunity to prove it.

Still, there is, I believe, an extraordinary saying involving a fat lady and a good deal of singing, and, calling at least the gist of it to mind, I resisted the impulse to shrivel up and die and instead apologised humbly for the misunderstanding and maintained what I hoped was my brightest, most worthy, expression until I was the other side of the heavy oak door.

And then I shrivelled up and died.

Fortunately it's very hard to stay shrivelled for long in the company of people who 'twinkle'. As if by magic, within moments of being bundled into Dr Mason's waiting car I was actually quite looking forward to lunch. All that shrivelling gives one an appetite. Yumm.

In fact, lunch was to be taken 'In Hall' with the rest of the college and thus was no less daunting a prospect than the rest of my schedule. I was acutely conscious of my wig and not, I feel, unduly concerned that a freak hurricane might pass through the building at any moment and take my hair with it. But I was hungry and curious, possibly the two most powerful of human instincts (after love, naturally), and sure enough one o'clock found me taking my place at table.

The hall was vast, with long trestle tables stretching down towards a raised platform. From one corner presided a gleaming grand piano and, over all, the variously austere, uncomfortable, beaming and proud faces of former college luminaries cast their worthy gaze, forever immortalised in oil and canvas. The food, it transpired, was unmemorable but the company was warm, relaxed and entertaining and served to further my instinct that this was indeed where I belonged. Sitting there amongst that happy, animated throng, the dark underworld which had held me captive for so long was as a long-ago dream, as far from my own reality as it was from that of the young faces around me. My spirit, far from having been crushed by the weight of the past nine months, sat up and shook itself, as a dog shaking water droplets from its shaggy coat, and entered in to the lively fray, delighting in its new-found freedom. It seemed I hadn't forgotten! I still remembered how to live in this world where the sun was always there, even if you couldn't see it, and the night sky really was black with tiny pin-pricks of stars, where tears could be for joy as well as sadness - and I wasn't going to die tomorrow...

Well, I reasoned, if I wasn't going to die tomorrow then

I had better make the most of today – and at this point that meant specifically my third and final interview. My last assignation, I had been assured by Dr Mason, would be my most relaxed; and since it was with him, I felt that on the whole he was in a pretty strong position to judge. This comfortable scenario, however, was not insignificantly ruffled by the fact that the college principal, whom I was yet to meet, would also be in – very official – attendance. Still, the setting was congenial, Dr Mason's storybook drawing-room in his storybook cottage for storybook tea and cakes, and I had to confess that it was not many minutes after having curled into his storybook sofa before I was feeling decidedly at ease. The Principal, Dr Fiddes, was actually rather like a character from a storybook himself – a 'Lord of the Rings-ish' kind of a book – and utterly courteous and charming. A renowned – and not a little controversial – Professor of Theology, he was keen to explore my own attitudes to faith and Christianity, and the conversation flowed freely and naturally.

And then they asked me.

"And what have you been reading over the past year?" Dr Fiddes enquired with interest.

Sitting there with a steaming cup of tea in my hand and such convivial faces on either side, I just couldn't do it. I was all out of bluff. "Well," I began, "having been in hospital for most of the year, the only books I have really been able to tackle with zeal are crime novels. I don't suppose you have read any Agatha Christie?"

And then an extraordinary thing happened. God came down and worked a miracle, right there under our noses, and I knew all over again that life was truly a wondrous thing.

"As it happens," Dr Fiddes replied, "my hobby is crime fiction. How do you think Agatha Christie compares with Colin Dexter?"

And we were away. And I never looked back. And who knows, next time I see him I might even ask him what he thinks of 'Five on a Treasure Island'…

Chapter Forty
Poop! Poop!

It was when we were on the journey home that it really hit me.

Mummy had met me, as arranged, at the Wykeham Tea Rooms just opposite New College, a favourite 'toasted cheese sandwich' sort of a place for my brother Timmy on his way back to choir school each term. Fortunately, such was her relief at seeing me returned in one piece that it more than compensated for her motherly consternation at finding me outside said tea rooms in enthusiastic embrace with an unknown man at least three times my age. "But I just couldn't help it," I explained, not very reassuringly, "Rex, (Dr Mason), is just such a lovely man."

Still, gamely suppressing her mild anxiety that in proudly waving me off to university next year she might well be opening up a whole new can of worms, Mummy listened animatedly to my excited babble as I recounted the day's adventures.

And suddenly I realised. More than anything in the world I wanted to go to Oxford University. As I relived my day; the glorious rush of intellectual challenge; the bright, lively comradeship amongst the students; the chance to set out on a new and unknown path and the exciting, even thrilling, prospect of rediscovered independence, I knew without a doubt that I belonged.

And I had surely blown it. In a single moment of melodramatic over-sensitivity I had 'scuppered' my chances; it might as well have been Fate that I had shaken a metaphorical fist at and My Future that lay behind the proud oak door as I closed it heavy-hearted behind me. Tired, emotional and sad, I burst into tears and Mummy took me home.

Almost as we were walking through the door the telephone rang. It was Ruth, a friend and 'mentor', whose influence – she having two years previously graduated from Regents Park College with a First in English Language and Literature – was paramount in our decision to apply to the University. Keen to know how things had gone, she listened intently as I poured out my woes. And then she chuckled. At this, even more curious than I was put out, I paused for a moment and gave her an opportunity to expand on her inappropriate response.

"You're in!" she grinned down the wire. "He loves someone who's a bit feisty – congratulations!"

If I wasn't altogether persuaded by her conviction, the call that came through just moments later left no room for doubt.

So there I lay, sprawled on the old wooden floorboards – rich and warm beneath me with countless years of love and wax and the worn, soft remembering of countless feet passing down the ages and across that wide, bright landing that snaked out above the stairs – and replaced the telephone back on its, firmly 20th century, nest. And I smiled.

He wasn't supposed to call, Dr Mason had said. We were supposed to wait for the official letters to go out in a few weeks time. But he had wanted me to know as soon as possible.

As I bounded down the wide red staircase towards the kitchen, the news swelling in my chest and the joyful tears streaming down my face, I stretched out my arms and they were wings. And, as my feet began to lift from the ground, the long-recalled words resounded through my heart and soul;

"Look out world, I'm on my way!"

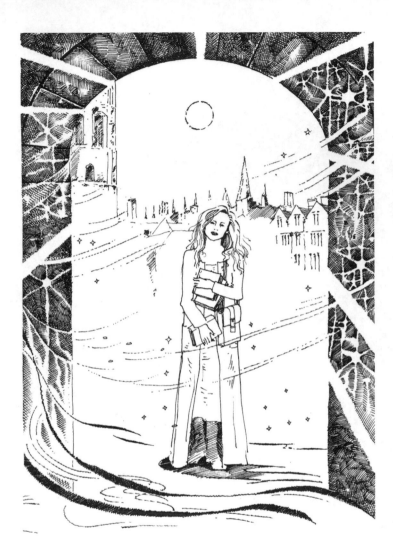

""'Look out world, I'm on my way!'""

Chapter Forty One
The beginning

And so I was.

Epilogue

So, here I am, and through another attic bedroom window the early evening sunlight pours, casting its still intense light across the pale, whitewashed floorboards. And the end, you see, really was just the beginning and, as the birds serenade me out of another day, I know that tomorrow too the world and I will wake and start all over again. But because of today we will be just a little changed. The grass will be a fraction longer, the buds a little fatter, eggs will be a little closer to hatching and I, well I will be one step further on my journey, if not towards nirvana then perhaps a little closer to understanding what it's all about.

The story I have told you is about a year in my life; an extraordinary year in which my attitudes to that life, to my faith and to the world around me, were altered forever. But it is also about the ten years that have followed. It is about an ever flowing stream of consciousness and growth that has for its source an extraordinary window of time, that has become, through those years, a part of the living, breathing 'quixoticness' that is me.

What happened to me twelve years ago, at the very point at which I was stepping out over the threshold of life is, for now, just as I have told you. Perhaps if I had told you then it might not have been the same story. And if I tell you once more when I am eighty-five I hope that, through the fullness of life and experience, it will be a different story all over again. Such is the wonderful fickleness of Memory.

Perhaps then, in part, this book is a celebration of Memory: a homage to the extraordinary ability that, with a little patience and faith and a whole lot of love, the human mind has to take adversity and mould and shape it to become a positive part of an ever changing spirit...

And it is too a celebration of life's journey; of the twists and turns that face one on one's path; of chance, coincidence, opportunity and 'fate'; and of whatever it is that lies just around that next bend. My life is still extraordinary, not least because it is still mine to be lived. And when it comes down to life's eternal mysteries, there's only one thing of which I can really be sure: as long as there are still corners, then there can be no doubt that I am still on the road!

Poop! Poop!

Postcript

Alchemy

Emma's arrival at Oxford was electric. I knew, within moments, that I would have to marry her at all costs.

What a contrast to expectations! We had all known, of course, that the new year of English Lit students would include a sick girl, part way through her cancer treatment. But the girl who walked through the door at the start of the Michaelmas term was no 'sick girl'. She was a life-force. The languid, hazed torpor of those students days was suddenly illuminated by the dash of cape and hat, the brilliant insight of mind alight with eager curiosity, the grace of form and the flash of eye that set us all hoping.

Coming face to face with this determination to conquer adversity and live life to its limit, changed the course of those years for many of us. Emma showed me then the value of Doing at a time when I was sinking in the murky art of Not Doing. Visiting her in hospital on one of her occasional stays, I found her dictating an essay that a year before I had gone to lengths to avoid undertaking. Admiration. Inspiration. Awe.

Within the year, I had secured my own triumph. Emma agreed to marry me and Coleridge and Henry James became part of our plan for the next years before London and the world opened before us.

And every month and year that has passed since then has reaffirmed that initial wonder and admiration. Twelve years on Emma is, physically, badly weakened by the drugs and radiotherapy that saved her. She suffers near constant pain and the restrictions on her life increase as time passes. Yet, while I snarl my way homewards, weary after work, I know I will once again soon be face to face with the life-force-girl, brimming with excitement over the tiniest detail of nature, the faintest whisper of hope on the wind. The house is full of angels and those vanquished demons quail at the sound of laughter and the light of hope that Emma has filled her cup with. To overflowing........

Lorenzo Romanelli – 28th March 2004

Appendix

Amy's Poem

"I wish I was a little clown
As sweet and good as gold.
And if I was a little clown
You, in my arms, could hold.

When things begin to get you down
I'll cuddle you up tight
And tell you from your little clown
That everything's alright."

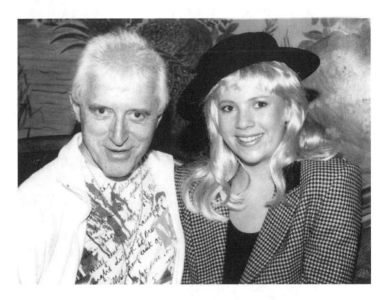

Emma with Sir. Jimmy Saville O.B.E.

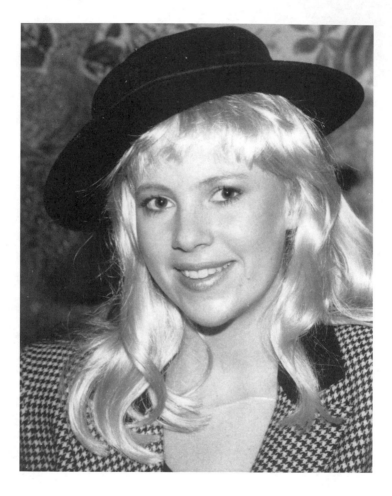

Emma with a fine head of the Duchess's hair.

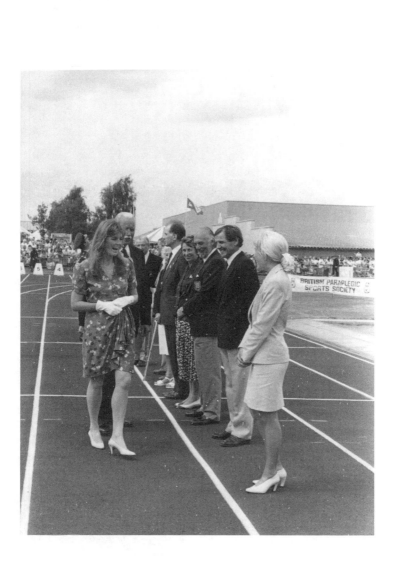

Emma meets her friend, the Duchess of York.

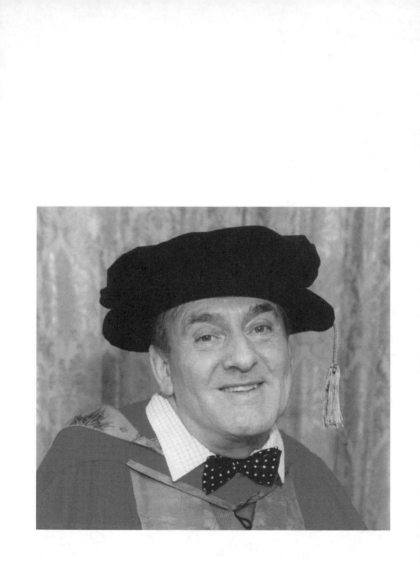

Dr. Michael Rogers - © The Bucks Herald

Wingrave Revisited

Emma has been my friend for many years. I first grew to know her at Wingrave Combined School, where she was one of the youngest by far of my class of eleven and twelve year olds. She was a delight to teach, so responsive and keen, with an absolute passion for words. I soon realised that she had enormous literary potential. Under her leadership as 'editor', the class won a major Bucks Herald competition with a prize of £250, with which the school acquired its first computer. Seven years later I heard of her dreadful illness, and sent her, for comfort, a large woolly black lamb to cuddle! And from then, our correspondence began, and has continued to this day.

Later, when she gained a place at Oxford, she invited me for the day – something I much appreciated. Wearing a flattering golden wig, she gave me an interesting tour of the college. We had lunch, and best of all we chatted, Emma again so excited and vivacious. She was obviously living her life to the full: despite her serious physical problems, enjoying every minute, eagerly lapping up everything university had to offer.

Over the years I have received amazing letters, which I shall always treasure. Soon 'Dear Mr & Mrs Morley' changed to 'Margaret & Ken'. Her messages were so bright and loving, with never ever, ever, any complaint, but joy in all the little things of life that many of us busy, bustling people never even notice. From her bedroom window or walking through her magic 'little wood', she writes so eloquently of the changing seasons, the colours and the beauty all around.

We wish brave Emma every success in this, her big new adventure. She certainly deserves it.

Margaret Morley
June 26th 2004

The Bucks Herald

ESTABLISHED 1832
PROPRIETORS: G. T. DE FRAINE (1973) LTD.
LONDON OFFICE: ARTHUR CLAY
80 FLEET STREET, EC4Y 1EL. TEL. 583 7000

Registered Office: 2/4 Exchange Street, Aylesbury, Bucks, HP20 1UJ. Place of Registration — London. Registered Number 1144980

EXCHANGE STREET - AYLESBURY - TELEPHONE 24444

July 14, 1982.

Dear Emma,

I thought you might like this picture. It's a good photograph of at least one of us!

I really enjoyed working with you and your team.

Yours sincerely,

Editor.

Under Emma's leadership as 'editor', the class won a major Bucks Herald competition.

212

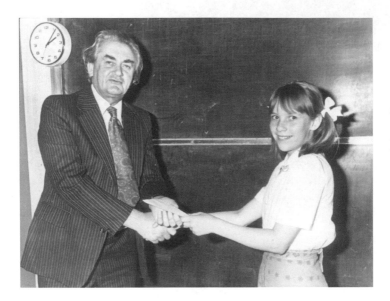

Emma with former Bucks Herald editor Phil Fountain.

About;
Teenage Cancer Trust

This amazing story, written so eloquently by this exceptionally talented young woman, embodies so much of the spirit of what Teenage Cancer Trust is trying to achieve. Emma is a born fighter who has battled against her illness and the effects of its treatment. Through the tapestry of her words she sends a positive message to us all about what really are the important things in life. This book is a good read in its own right, not just because of its subject matter. But the compelling combination of the two is what really sets it apart.

And to top all that Emma has decided to donate a very significant percentage of the proceeds from the book to Teenage Cancer Trust so that youngsters in the future can benefit from improved services and treatment. This donation will enable us to develop more units around the country that are specifically geared towards teenagers. Environments that whilst providing the best possible care also include computers, Playstations, social facilities and are geared especially to the needs of young people. It will also help us to deliver our associated support services for families and our education and awareness programme in schools and universities throughout the country. (www.teencancer.org)

Thank you Emma for your selfless generosity.

Thanks too to Tim at Next Century Books who has helped to bring this venture into the linelight that it richly deserves.

Simon Davies
Chief Executive Officer
Teenage Cancer Trust
June 29, 2004

Stoke Mandeville
HOSPITAL NHS TRUST

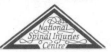

Mandeville Road
Aylesbury
Buckinghamshire
HP21 8AL
Tel: 01296 315000

I first met EMMA when she was lying on top of a bed, in an oyster satin nightie. She was dying - so we all set to work.

The Hospital did its bit, Emma did her bit and I did mine.

We won, Death lost and this book is her story. Read it and if your back is ever pressed against the wall of life – read it again, it could fill you with fight when you might just need it.

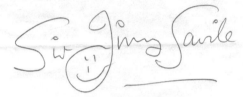

Sir Jimmy Savile, OBE KCSG LL.D F.CYB

SM

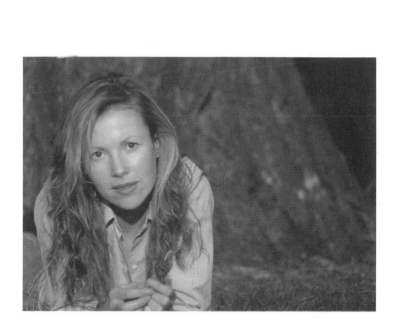

Emma Bowes Romanelli - April 2004